A Victim No More:
Overcoming
Irritable
Bowel
Syndrome

Safe, Effective Therapies for Relief from Bowel Complaints

JONATHAN M. BERKOWITZ, M.D.

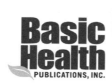

Basic
Health
PUBLICATIONS, INC.

D0376963

Basic Health Publications, Inc.
28812 Top of the World Drive
Laguna Beach, CA 92651
949-715-7327

Library of Congress Cataloging-in-Publication Data
Berkowitz, Jonathan M.
    A victim no more : overcoming irritable bowel syndrome / Jonathan M. Berkowitz.
       p. cm.
Includes bibliographical references and index.
    ISBN 10: 1-59120-078-4
    ISBN 13: 978-1-59120-078-9
    1. Irritable colon—Popular works. I. Title.
    RC862.I77B47   2003
    616.3'42—dc21
                                        2003008650

Editor: John Anderson
Typesetter/Book design: Gary A. Rosenberg
Cover design: Mike Stromberg

Printed in the United States of America

10   9   8   7   6   5   4   3

Contents

To Paul G.
for Your
Faith and
Kindness

Introduction

There is little doubt that irritable bowel syndrome (IBS) is one of the most challenging disorders for both the patient and healthcare professional. The same can be said about authoring a book on IBS—this work has been one of my most challenging in nearly twenty years of writing. IBS is a complex syndrome with multiple clinical presentations. While many factors contribute to IBS, in its simplest terms, IBS is a disorder characterized by altered bowel motility and hypersensitivity. This results in a constellation of symptoms that typically includes abdominal pain, diarrhea, constipation, and bloating. Yet, ask any person who suffers from IBS, and you will quickly learn that such simple distillations are never possible. Symptoms vary widely between individuals and even in the same person. And while there are specific symptoms one must have in order to be diagnosed with IBS, the range of possible associated symptoms is legion.

The controversy surrounding IBS stems from the confusing and often conflicting scientific literature. We are, however, coming closer to understanding this syndrome and have witnessed a quantum leap in the way physicians and researchers think about IBS. Known as the Brain-Gut Model, this theory postulates that the physical and psychological manifestations of IBS occur as a result of a complex interplay between the central nervous system and the bowel's own enteric nervous system. While the Brain-Gut Model has revolutionized how we think about IBS, researchers still must grapple with the contributions that diet, allergies, and emotions make to this syndrome. Despite fifty years of intense investigation, IBS remains one of the most difficult syndromes for the physician to tackle, and we still have far more questions than answers.

I'm a firm believer that knowledge is power—the more you know about IBS, the better you will feel. This is why the first chapters of this book are devoted to understanding how the gastrointestinal system normally works and how IBS affects this system. Chapters 1 and 2 also provide a comprehensive review of abnormal bowel function, with an extensive discussion of diarrhea and constipation, two cardinal IBS symptoms. These chapters also illustrate the complexity of IBS, a condition frequently characterized by nonspecific symptoms that can be related to multiple disorders. It is this nonspecificity of symptoms that makes IBS especially challenging for healthcare professionals and patients alike.

It is this confusing symptom complex that in the past has led to extensive and, at times, excessive diagnostic evaluations. But our increased understanding of IBS has allowed the medical profession to standardize diagnostic protocols, the subject of Chapter 3. Chapter 3 details what you can expect during a traditional medical evaluation, explaining the basic diagnostic tests. Furthermore, as any healthcare professional will tell you, a detailed history is critical to arriving at the correct diagnosis: Chapter 3 provides those vital questions you should ask to achieve a better understanding of your body and IBS.

One of the most important lessons of this book is that IBS represents a complex interplay between mind and body. For decades, many physicians and patients mistakenly believed that IBS was primarily a psychological disorder, a belief that resulted in many people being told that IBS was "all in their head." Let it be said that nothing could be further from the truth, as researchers have consistently described multiple physiological abnormalities in IBS. Conversely, mind-body interactions are a rapidly emerging and legitimate field of medicine, and we now appreciate that disorders such as asthma, fibromyalgia, and even heart disease are impacted tremendously by how we think and feel. The same is true of IBS—we cannot ignore its complex mind-body interactions. Therefore, Chapter 4 is devoted to the psychology of IBS.

Modern medicine is finally realizing that health is truly a partnership between doctor and patient. We now know that the best outcomes occur when people take responsibility for their health. Physicians and patients understand that what we eat and how we live dramatically impact our health. Chapter 5 examines diet and IBS, offering several dietary modifications that can help relieve symptoms. Chapter 6 reviews vitamin, mineral, and herbal IBS therapies, and Chapter 7 offers a review of alternative treatments, such as acupuncture, cognitive-behavioral therapy, and hypnotherapy. Chapter 8 explores the impact that lifestyle has on the bowel, especially exercise on IBS.

Finally, Chapter 9 offers a brief review of conventional pharmacologic IBS management. As the reader will learn, one of the distinguishing features of this book is that no therapy or recommendation is offered without reasonable support in the scientific literature for its use, with key references listed in the back leading to additional reading.

While there is no single magic herb, drug, vitamin, or mineral that cures IBS, you will learn that IBS can be controlled and even beaten. As with most conditions, the best outcomes result from individualized treatment that takes the entire person into consideration. This is especially true for IBS, as no two people with this syndrome have exactly the same causes or symptoms. Because IBS varies widely from person to person, some trial and error is often needed before arriving at a satisfactory strategy, a natural reflection of how different individuals uniquely react to specific therapies. In other words, what works for someone else may not work for you. This is why I encourage you to try different therapies: Some people may find that dietary modifications are most effective, while others may learn that a particular supplement or herb works best. By asking yourself the right questions and finding those therapies that work best for you, I hope you will not only be able to better control your symptoms but also one day eliminate IBS from your life.

Chapter 1

What Is IBS?

Man should strive to have his intestines relaxed
all the days of his life.
—MOSES MAIMONIDES

Julie sat on the edge of my examining table. "Doctor," she began with a heavy sigh, "I can't even make dinner plans anymore—my life has become a mess. I never know when I'm going to have to run to the bathroom—and even worse, when I have to go, I really have to go. Stop right there, pull over at the next gas station, get up from the table—whatever. And the pain, the gas, is awful." Julie, trying not to cry, continued, "I've been to three doctors, and they all told me something different—I just want to know what's wrong and get things back to normal. I just want to get my life back."

Such is the typical story I hear when listening to someone who has irritable bowel syndrome (IBS). Yet, what is IBS? This is a question that has plagued physicians for decades. Is IBS an organic disorder or a psychological problem? Does IBS share features of both? Over the years, there has been tremendous confusion over the meaning of IBS, with opinions differing among physicians and patients alike. This confusion is reflected in the various names given to what we now call IBS: irritable colon syndrome, spastic colitis, nervous colon, and mucous colitis.

The good news is that after years of intensive research, even though many questions remain, we are finally getting some important answers. What has emerged is that IBS is a constellation of conditions that shares similar, but at times distinct, features. It turns out that many roads lead to the syndrome we now call IBS. Perhaps one of the most profound discoveries regarding IBS relates to the complex interplay between the central nervous system and the bowel's own nervous system. Known as the "Brain-Gut Model" and the focus of Chapter 4, this concept of reciprocal interaction has enabled us to better decipher the mind-body interactions often observed in people with IBS.

What we can say with certainty is that IBS at the most fundamental level represents a state of dysfunctional bowel motility that involves the entire bowel, from small intestine to rectum. IBS is also characterized by visceral (bowel) hypersensitivity, so that people with IBS are more sensitive to stimuli originating from their bowel. How these derangements translate into symptoms will vary from individual to individual; however, the vast majority of people who suffer from IBS complain of altered bowel habits coupled with abdominal pain, with varying degrees of diarrhea and constipation.

As distressing as these symptoms may be, rest assured that no one has ever died from IBS. Equally important, IBS does not reduce one's life span or increase the risk of developing a serious disorder like cancer or inflammatory bowel disease.

With respect to treatment, you will learn that IBS can be managed and even overcome. From a purely statistical perspective, the prognosis for people with IBS is excellent. One study found that 85 percent of those afflicted will improve with first-line medical therapy. Clearly, it is reasonable to expect that you should lead a normal, active, and healthy life—the life each of us so richly deserves.

WHY IBS?

It is human nature to ask "why?" And with IBS, this is a question that continues to undergo intense scrutiny. In this chapter, we will review both normal and abnormal bowel function, concentrating on IBS-related findings. Many authorities used to believe that IBS was primarily a psychological problem that had no organic or physiological basis. Today, while psychology clearly plays a role in some people with IBS, we are learning that the bowels of people with IBS are clearly different from normal bowels. As you read this chapter, it will become apparent that many variations of bowel function have been reported in IBS patients that distinguish them from people who do not have IBS. Not all of these findings are operative in each and every patient with IBS, and what has emerged is that IBS is a heterogeneous disorder, with no two people with IBS being exactly alike. In other words, while there are many different types of bowel dysfunction found in IBS, not every person with IBS will display the same findings when examined.

We still have many more questions about IBS than we have answers, and the multitude of findings described in this book adds weight to the statement "The more you know, the less you know." Despite all of the conflicting and confusing findings, we can say with reasonable certainty that IBS is a disorder characterized by "psychosocial factors, altered motility, and/or heightened sensory function." How all these findings translate into this syndrome, and how much of what we see in IBS is truly abnormal versus a simple variant of normal, is the subject of ongoing research.

Yet, we are still at a loss to give an adequate explanation of why people get IBS. What can be said with reasonable certainty is that the condition probably results from a complex interplay between genes and environment: We may find that in some people genes are more responsible, whereas in others environment plays a larger role. Many theories have been put forth regarding the question of "why?"—most with an element of truth. For some people, the cause of IBS is related to a food allergy. For others, inflammation from a prior infection may be to blame. Still others may have psychological issues that are responsible for their symptoms. It is doubtful that a single universal answer can be identified as the cause of IBS, and what is emerging from the scientific literature is that IBS is a very individual syndrome, with different processes operating in different individuals.

This variability has profound ramifications for the diagnosis and management of IBS. As you will learn in the following chapters, the diagnosis and treatment of IBS can be as varied as the many suspected causes. And, as will be emphasized throughout this book, an individualized approach to the management of IBS has consistently produced the best results.

WHO HAS IBS?

IBS is a common condition, and studies have found that 15 to 20 percent of the population may be afflicted. In fact, IBS is the most common reason for referring a patient to a gastroenterologist, responsible for 20 to 50 percent of all specialist referrals. The most common diagnosis made by - gastroenterologists in America, IBS is responsible for approximately 12 percent of primary care visits. IBS is also the second most frequent reason for missing work. (Number one is the common cold.)

Despite these impressive numbers, most experts believe that the number of individuals with IBS is underestimated, as a significant subgroup of people with IBS may never seek medical attention. In fact, studies estimate that only 25 percent of those afflicted actually seek medical care. The reasons behind this finding are complex and in part relate to how people interpret their symptoms and decide when to seek help. Also, some individuals with IBS have had their symptoms for so long that they consider their bowel habits normal, not even realizing they have the disorder.

Women have IBS three times more often than men. This finding, however, may be distorted by health-seeking behavior and referral patterns, since some authorities suspect that IBS affects men and women equally, but women are more likely to visit a physician. IBS is more common in North America and Europe, with lower rates reported in Asia and Africa. The reasons behind this geographic variability are complex, but it is speculated that this reflects cultural differences in health-seeking behavior.

In addition, IBS has a tremendous impact on our healthcare system: It is estimated that IBS treatment costs in the United States total $8 billion annually, with another $25 billion in indirect costs.

WHAT ARE THE RISK FACTORS?

There are no established risk factors for IBS, and the condition most likely results from an interplay among genes, environment, and childhood experiences. While the risk factors for IBS remain ill-defined, a particularly disturbing finding is that people with IBS are more likely to have a history of physical and sexual abuse. Approximately 32 percent of those with IBS report a history of physical abuse, and 44 percent report a history of sexual abuse. These statistics may be particularly alarming to some of you reading this book. Let it be said right here that physical and sexual abuse has everything to do with the perpetrator through no fault of the victim. For individuals who have been through these regrettable ordeals, there is help available, a subject discussed in more detail in Chapter 4. Other traumatic events have also been associated with IBS, and several studies demonstrate that IBS onset in some individuals closely parallels and may be triggered by a traumatic emotional experience.

While IBS has no impact on longevity, it does put people at risk for fibromyalgia, migraine headache, chronic pelvic pain, chronic fatigue, noncardiac chest pain, and interstitial cystitis. Fibromyalgia is a medical condition involving widespread musculoskeletal pain and stiffness, which is often accompanied by poor sleep and chronic fatigue. Interstitial cystitis is a painful chronic bladder condition that causes symptoms similar to those found in a urinary tract infection but without evidence of infection.

WHAT CAUSES IBS?

A major obstacle in understanding IBS is that despite five decades of intensive research, we have been unable to identify any anatomic, microscopic, infectious, or biochemical derangement that adequately accounts for the syndrome. Multiple theories have been put forth to explain IBS. Some authorities suggest that certain people are genetically "predisposed" to IBS, with the syndrome "triggered" by an infection, drug (antibiotic), abdominal surgery, or emotional trauma. Dietary factors are blamed in some individuals, with suspects ranging from a low-fiber diet to food allergies to lactose intolerance (discussed in Chapter 5). Alcohol and tobacco abuse remain suspect, as does aerophagia (a fancy word for swallowing air) induced by anxiety. Hyperventilation is another mechanism proposed to play a role in IBS. A variety of chemical mediators like gastrin and cholecystokinin have been associated with IBS, but their true relationship remains elusive.

Infection has also been blamed, and some experts suspect that inflammatory changes resulting from a previous bowel infection may trigger the syndrome. Authorities have suspected since the 1950s that IBS may be an inflammatory disorder. While we are only beginning to understand the role of inflammation in the disease, several studies have found that the bowel mucosa and nerves may be inflamed in IBS. This inflammation, while not as profound as in inflammatory bowel disease, may ultimately be found to play an important role in IBS. Infection appears to be the most likely culprit for this inflammation, and a bowel infection that occurs during a time of severe emotional stress appears to be an especially potent combination that may initially trigger IBS. This may help explain why some people first develop IBS during periods of psychological trauma. It is also theorized that inflammation may activate peripheral sensitization or hypermotility, thereby resulting in the visceral hypersensitivity and altered gut motility characteristic of IBS. In other words, the inflammation can make the bowel's nerves ultrasensitive to stimuli and change how the bowel moves.

Others suspect that alterations in the microorganisms that normally inhabit the bowel are the cause of IBS. This has led some researchers to treat IBS with probiotics, a subject covered in Chapter 5.

Authorities have also suggested that, in some women, IBS may be related to a gynecological disorder. As any woman can tell you, menstruation is not one of their favorite pastimes, and this is especially true for women with IBS. Several studies have found that women tend to experience more IBS-related symptoms when menstruating. While the mechanisms behind this need to be determined, it is suspected that chemical imbalances are to blame.

One of the most promising avenues of research relates to emerging evidence that IBS is probably caused by dysfunctional interactions between nerves and neurotransmitters. Nerve cells, or neurons, communicate with one another through chemicals called neurotransmitters. One of the major neurotransmitters found in the gut is serotonin, the same chemical found in the brain that is associated with depression. Serotonin is an important chemical messenger that is in part responsible for symptoms like abdominal pain, bloating, nausea, vomiting, and bowel contraction. While research on serotonin and IBS is still in its infancy, several studies have found that people with IBS have elevated levels of serotonin in their blood and bowel.

We will discuss these theories in later chapters. What is important to understand now from this bewildering array of conjectures is that each of these theories may contain an element of truth that can be found in some, but not all, individuals with IBS. But the fact remains that when we attempt to say what "causes" irritable bowel syndrome, we still have many more questions than answers. While we clearly need to learn more about IBS, today we are closer than ever to understanding the mechanisms behind this syndrome.

Exciting new advances in our understanding of neurobiology has led to the Brain-Gut Model of IBS. Central to this model are the ways the central nervous system (CNS) and the bowel's own nervous system, the enteric nervous system (ENS), communicate. This model has revolutionized the way we think about IBS and, for the first time, offers a unifying framework that begins to explain many of the mind-body interactions observed in this syndrome. While we will explore this topic in detail in Chapter 4, in its simplest terms, the Brain-Gut Model describes IBS as the consequence of dysfunctional communication between the CNS and ENS. This communication takes place through nerve impulses and chemicals that establish a vicious "fear" cycle, which ultimately translates into the constellations of symptoms we associate with IBS.

NORMAL BOWEL FUNCTION

Before we can discuss the symptoms of IBS and understand abnormal bowel function, it will be instructive to review how the bowel works normally. The gastrointestinal tract essentially represents a long tube that runs from one end of the body to the other. At its superior or proximal end is the mouth, with the primary function of ingesting and preparing food for entry into the stomach. At the risk of stating the obvious, this is achieved by inserting food into the mouth and using the teeth to break this food into more digestible pieces. With the exception of a small amount of digestive enzymes present in the salvia, the majority of digestion begins in the stomach and continues through the small and large intestines.

Once the food has been sufficiently chewed, it is swallowed into the esophagus, which, through a series of muscular contractions, propels the food bolus into the stomach. It is in the stomach that most of the work of breaking down food occurs. In addition to the churning action caused by contraction and relaxation of the stomach's muscles, a process known as peristalsis, the stomach contains digestive chemicals, such as hydrochloric acid, and enzymes that accelerate digestion.

Helping to move and mix this partially digested food is water that is secreted into the stomach. Large fluid shifts occur during digestion, with an average nine liters of fluid entering the intestines daily, but only one liter of fluid ever reaching the colon. Equally dramatic, the average daily fluid load that is actually passed in the stool is only approximately 0.2 liters, a testimony to the reabsorbing capacity of the large intestine. In fact, many bowel disorders are directly related to imbalances between the bowel's secretion of water and how poorly this water is reabsorbed.

The stomach has two ends: the gastroesophageal junction, which relaxes to permit food from the esophagus to enter the stomach, and the pylorus, which permits food to pass from the stomach to the small intestine. Before we discuss the small intestine, let's quickly examine what digestion is all about.

Inside the bowel, food can only be absorbed at the molecular level. For instance, a meat and potato dinner gets broken down into smaller and smaller pieces of food by the mouth and the stomach. By the time this meal knocks on the door of the pylorus, it has the consistency of a fine slurry. This slurry is further broken down in the small intestine by digestive enzymes that reduce these fine food particles into the molecules of digestion. Specifically, these molecules are proteins, fats, and sugars (carbo-hydrates). The mashing and bashing, however, don't end here. Proteins are further broken down into digestible amino acids, and carbohydrates are digested into sugars, such as glucose. In general, it is only when proteins are reduced to amino acids and carbohydrates broken down into individual sugars that true digestion can occur, as these molecules are absorbed into the bloodstream for delivery to the body's cells.

THE SMALL INTESTINE

The pylorus is the gatekeeper between the stomach and the small intestine and is very picky as to what will be allowed through, like a bouncer at a very exclusive club: If food particles are not small enough, they will not pass through the pylorus and into the small intestine. The small intestine is divided into three parts: the duodenum, the jejunum, and the ileum. The chief function of the small intestine is to digest and absorb molecular food particles while secreting and absorbing water and electrolytes. The first part of the small intestine is the duodenum, and it is here that pancreatic and biliary digestive enzymes are mixed with the partially digested slurry to further enhance digestion and absorption.

Like the rest of the gastrointestinal tract, the small intestine employs peristalsis to move food along its length. Peristalsis is especially active after ingesting a meal. There is a special type of smooth-muscle peristalsis unique to the small bowel called the migrating motor complex (MMC), which primarily serves to clear waste products from the small intestine. The MMC is also predictable, lasting approximately four minutes and occurring every sixty to ninety minutes.

Once the food has been broken down into its molecular components, it can be transported across the lining of the small intestine and into the bloodstream. Once in the bloodstream, these molecules are used to make energy, proteins, sugars, and fat. While digestion primarily occurs in the stomach and duodenum, the absorption of food molecules primarily occurs in the jejunum and ileum. This leaves the large bowel or colon with the job of dealing with the waste products of digestion.

The small and large intestines are also divided into layers. The bowel is essentially a hollow collapsible tube that is lined by mucosal tissue known as intestinal epithelium. It is at this mucosal interface that most of the work of digestion and absorption occurs. It is the mucosa that secretes water and electrolytes into the bowel and absorbs the molecules of digestion, which are then transported across the mucosal membrane on their way into the bloodstream. Once these molecules pass through the mucosa, they enter the submucosa, which contains the blood vessels that will transport these molecules to the rest of the body.

The submucosa is surrounded by layers of smooth muscle responsible for contracting and propelling the digested slurry of food and water through the small and large intestines. We are usually not aware of peristalsis; however, if peristalsis is particularly strong, we can experience it as an abdominal pain or cramp. Peristalsis is also the mechanism behind the sounds our stomachs occasionally make.

Finally, the bowel is bundled up by a tough sheath called the adventitia, which is in turn attached to various parts of the abdominal wall, keeping the bowels secured in place. Fixing the bowel to the abdominal wall is very important since bowels are soft, floppy structures that, if not positioned correctly, can twist and turn on themselves, potentially causing a dangerous obstruction. Also covering the anterior bowel is an apron of fatty tissue called the omentum. The omentum helps keep the bowel in place and also acts as a shield that can isolate diseased parts of the abdomen, such as the gallbladder, thereby protecting healthy structures.

THE LARGE INTESTINE

The large intestine is charged with absorption of water and electrolytes. It is also in the large intestine that stool is formed. Derangements in large bowel motility or absorption can result in diarrhea or constipation. Likewise, changes in electrolyte secretion or absorption can cause diarrhea. Like the small intestine, the large bowel is divided into parts. At the most proximal end, the cecum is connected to the ileum (the last part of the small bowel that serves as a portal into the large bowel). From the cecum, waste products enter the ascending colon, followed by the transverse colon, where the stool becomes progressively dehydrated. The ascending colon lies on the right side of your body and heads upward toward the liver, where it connects with the transverse colon that travels horizontally across the abdomen in the direction of the spleen.

This connection between the ascending and transverse colon is known as the hepatic flexure and represents a ninety-degree turn in the bowel from the vertical ascending colon to the horizontal transverse colon. From the transverse colon, the relatively formed stool enters the descending colon on its way to the rectum. The descending colon lies on the left side

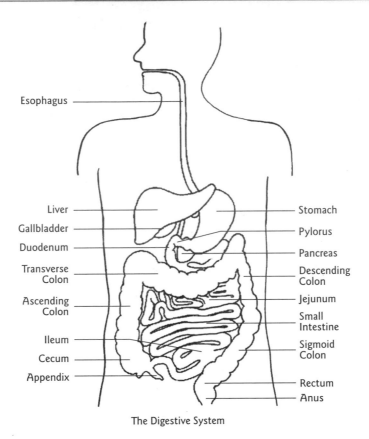

The Digestive System

of your body and propels the stool on its way to the rectum and anus. The junction between the transverse and descending colon is called the splenic flexure and, like the hepatic flexure, represents a ninety-degree turn in the bowel. The descending colon ultimately becomes the rectum and leads to the anus.

The primary functions of the ascending and transverse colon are to store stool and absorb water. Conversely, the descending colon's main purpose is to deliver stool to the rectum for expulsion through the anus. The rectum fundamentally serves as a storage site for feces prior to defecation. While the primary function of the large bowel is to absorb water and transport feces, a small amount of digestion and absorption does occur, primarily of carbohydrates by bacteria that normally live in the bowel.

It may surprise some of you to learn that you have bacteria making a home in your bowel; however, like many things in life, there are good and bad bacteria. You'll probably be even more surprised to learn that the average bowel contains more than 500 different types of bacteria. These bacteria rarely, if ever, cause problems and actually serve a useful purpose: Not only do these bacteria aid in food digestion, but they also help prevent potentially harmful bacteria from getting a foothold in the colon, multiplying, and causing disease. In fact, some antibiotics cause diarrhea because they alter the bowel's normal bacterial population. You can blame your bacteria on your parents and siblings, as the bowel is first colonized by bacteria during infancy and childhood, with the unique mix of gut flora determined by who you live with during the colonization period.

Besides being subject to standard peristaltic contractions, the large bowel has its own special type of muscular activity. Called the high-amplitude propagated contraction (HAPC), this contraction causes a large peristaltic wave that moves the entire colon, propelling colonic contents forward. Whereas peristalsis tends to be a local phenomenon, HAPCs are a colon-wide event, which usually occur five times daily, most commonly in the morning after awakening and after a meal. This is why most people have bowel movements in the morning after breakfast. Too many HAPCs may be a reason why some people have diarrhea. Also, like the small intestine, the colon has a background muscular "tone" upon which these HAPCs occur.

Most colonic motor activity is mediated by the autonomic nervous system, but hormones and gastrointestinal distention caused by ingested food also play major roles. Finally, while the bowel is active during the day, the same cannot be said when we are asleep. In people with or without IBS, the bowel is at rest when we sleep and this is the reason why people with IBS normally do not experience symptoms while asleep. Experts suspect that during sleep, the bowel is subject to less emotional and physiological input, thereby resulting in a "quiet" gut.

THE INTESTINAL NERVOUS SYSTEM

The small and large intestines are controlled by an intrinsic and extrinsic nervous system, which are both part of the ENS. The intrinsic nervous system is primarily responsible for controlling the involuntary smooth muscles of the bowel and the absorption and secretion of fluids and electrolytes. The extrinsic nervous system is part of the autonomic nervous system. The autonomic nervous system normally controls those bodily functions we don't usually have to think about, such as respiration, blood pressure, and heart rate. I emphasize the word "usually" because there are some people who can exert some control over their autonomic nervous systems or have a system that is more sensitive to external stimuli than expected.

The autonomic nervous system is divided into parasympathetic and sympathetic nervous branches. In general, the actions of the sympathetic and parasympathetic nervous systems tend to antagonize each other, being either inhibitory or stimulatory. The splitting of the autonomic nervous system into sympathetic and parasympathetic divisions is based anatomically on where a particular nerve exits the spinal cord. In the bowel, the parasympathetic system tends to deal with excitatory impulses, whereas the sympathetic system tends to be both inhibitory and excitatory. With respect to the small and large bowels, the extrinsic nervous system is important for both motor and sensory function. Sensory function relates to your ability to perceive what is going on in your bowel and is mediated by sympathetic and parasympathetic nerves. The parasympathetic system has an impact on colonic motor function, while the sympathetic nerves also play a role in motor function, providing excitatory input to sphincter muscles while inhibiting the rest of the musculature.

These discussions regarding the nervous control of the intestines are important not only because the ENS plays a central role in the control of normal bowel function, but also because we are learning that derangements in the bowel's nervous system play a pivotal role in IBS. In fact, there is a rapidly emerging body of literature that implicates imbalances between the ENS and CNS as being responsible for causing IBS. Even more important, it is becoming evident that the most effective therapies for IBS are those that reestablish a balance between the CNS and ENS.

Intimately related to these various nervous systems is the electrical activity that stimulates the bowel. Nerves are like the electrical wiring in your house: Wires are merely conduits of electricity, while the electricity does all the work. Bowel nerves only conduct the electrical signals that control the bowel, and it is these electrical impulses that make the bowel work. But unlike the wires in your home that are directly connected to an outlet, the nerves in the gut are not directly attached to the bowel. Rather, communication between nerve and bowel occurs through chemical messengers that are released from the nerve after an electrical impulse passes through the nerve.

In the normal bowel, there are two basic forms of electrical activity.

The first type is called the slow wave and depends on the movement of sodium through the smooth muscle cells of the bowel. Also known as the "basic electric rhythm" or the "electric control activity," this slow wave is normally found in the distal (terminal) colon and has a rate of about six cycles per minute. Studies have shown that this pattern is altered in people with IBS, but the significance of this finding remains to be determined.

The second type of electrical activity is called a "spike action potential" or an "electric response activity." Whereas the slow wave provides background electrical activity for the gut, spike action potentials often cause contractions. Also unlike the slow wave, spike action potentials are calcium dependent.

There is increasing evidence that the electrical activity responsible for controlling the bowel's smooth muscle contraction is distorted in people with IBS. In fact, pharmacologic management of IBS attempts to manipulate this electrical activity, especially the spike potentials, which can be either increased or decreased depending on the drug used. One of the electrical abnormalities seen in IBS relates to spike potentials. Eating normally causes a rapid rise in spike potentials that peak in thirty minutes and subside in fifty minutes. In IBS, this initial rise in spike activity is dampened for the first thirty minutes. Furthermore, unlike the normal electrical response that is characterized by decreasing spike activity after thirty minutes, people with IBS have increasing spike activity that ultimately peaks seventy to ninety minutes later. Like the differences found in slow wave, the exact implications of these findings are undergoing intense investigation.

DEFECATION

The rectum primarily serves as a repository for feces that are waiting to be expelled through the anus. Through a complicated series of voluntary and involuntary muscle contractions, defecation is achieved when the rectum expels the stool through the relaxed anus. The major muscle involved in defecation is the puborectalis muscle, which, in the resting state, forms a sling around the anorectal junction and prevents the inadvertent release of stool. With defecation, parasympathetic stimulation relaxes the puborectalis, thereby releasing tension and allowing the passage of stool. The anal sphincter acts as a gatekeeper between the anus and the outside world and is normally contracted, only relaxing to permit defecation. Defecation is further aided by contractions of the rectosigmoid muscles, which propel the stool forward as the external anal sphincter relaxes under voluntary control.

If needed, a voluntary slight increase in intra-abdominal pressure can also help expel the stool. This voluntary increase in pressure, known as the Valsalva maneuver (or commonly called straining), can range from a normal gentle push to excessive effort that can ultimately result in nerve and bowel damage.

Also playing a major role in defecation are the smooth involuntary muscles of the rectum and the voluntary skeletal muscles of the pelvic floor. These pelvic floor muscles will become especially important in the discussion of constipation.

Chapter 2

Symptoms of IBS

Irritable bowel syndrome is classically associated with altered bowel habits and abdominal pain. The altered bowel habits in IBS translate into diarrhea or constipation, often characterized by an alternating course of diarrhea and constipation. Other common symptoms include increased gas or flatulence, an urgent desire to defecate, and the passage of small stools with scant amounts of mucus. Based on the symptoms, IBS is traditionally divided into four major subcategories: abdominal pain–predominant, diarrhea-predominant, constipation-predominant, and alternating constipation-diarrhea–predominant. In other words, some people tend to have mostly constipation, others tend to have mostly diarrhea, and others have alternating constipation and diarrhea.

Symptoms, as a rule, are extremely variable between patients. While no two people with IBS have the same symptoms and symptoms can vary widely within the same individual, after a certain period of time most people with IBS establish a relatively predictable pattern of symptoms. These symptoms typically undergo periods of exacerbation and remission, with symptoms often precipitated by predictable triggers.

One of the major challenges in establishing a diagnosis of IBS is that many of these symptoms are vague and nonspecific. In addition, all of these symptoms can occasionally occur in people with normal bowel function and also are common in individuals with gastrointestinal disease. Nevertheless, despite the variable presentation of IBS, the vast majority of people afflicted by this disorder will complain of diarrhea and/or constipation coupled with intermittent or persistent abdominal pain. These symptoms can range from very mild to extremely severe and may occur frequently or only occasionally. The causes behind IBS-related abdominal pain remain ill defined; however, it is suspected that colonic spasm is often to blame. While IBS-related diarrhea is usually associated with abdominal pain, up to 20 percent of people with IBS have painless diarrhea, which can be a normal response to stress.

At a very minimum, altered bowel habits and abdominal pain are needed to make a diagnosis of IBS. Altered bowel habits would include a noticeable change in bowel habits: At some point in a person's life, there was an identifiable transition from having "normal" bowel habits to the abnormalities in IBS. While some people can pinpoint when this change occurred, others often cannot. Likewise, some studies have clearly demonstrated that, in some people, this change is associated with a traumatic life event, while for others no clearly defined precipitating emotional event can be identified. This change in bowel habits can occur at any time, but most people experience changes in adolescence or early adulthood.

Approximately 25 to 50 percent of people with IBS may complain of heartburn, nausea, and vomiting. Complaints of regurgitated stomach acid and general indigestion are also common. Many of these symptoms are similar to those found in gastroesophageal reflux disorder (GERD), a condition characterized by the entry of stomach contents into the esophagus. In fact, studies have shown that some people with IBS have abnormal esophageal contractions, a finding common in GERD. The possibility of GERD should always be considered in the individual with IBS who also has heartburn.

Another common complaint with IBS is that eating food increases symptoms. Indeed, studies have shown hypermotility of the bowel lasting fifty minutes or more following a meal in some people with IBS. Other gut motility abnormalities have also been described with respect to food ingestion. For instance, food-induced motor activity in the normal bowel usually decreases within fifty minutes of a meal, but in people with IBS, motor activity may actually increase. In fact, several studies have documented that the small intestine displays increased motility with meals, a finding that may be in part responsible for the pain associated with IBS. There is also evidence that IBS may reflect a motility disorder that affects the entire gastrointestinal tract, as abnormal motor activity has been described in the gallbladder and stomach. Whether or not these findings are part of a larger, previously undiagnosed disorder of the gastrointestinal tract, or simply an IBS variant, remains to be determined.

While most symptoms relate to the bowel, many people with IBS complain of urinary dysfunction. Complaints related to sexual function are also reported, mostly concerning decreased sexual drive and, in women, pain during intercourse. The fact that many of these findings relate to organs that are in part under the control of the autonomic nervous system has led some investigators to suspect that IBS may be a disorder of autonomic function. The autonomic nervous system controls bodily functions that we normally don't have to think about, like digestion and respiration. As we will learn in Chapter 4, such speculations are not far from the truth.

ALTERED BOWEL HABITS

Critical to a diagnosis of IBS is a change in bowel habits. In fact, if a physician can't document altered bowel habits, there can be no diagnosis of IBS. One of the challenges in documenting altered bowel habits, especially in those over age forty, is that these changes most frequently occur in adolescence or early adulthood. As a result, there are many people who don't even know they have IBS because they have had the same pattern of bowel dysfunction for years or decades, a pattern that they've come to accept as normal. What this means for the healthcare practitioner is that they will have to attempt to discover information regarding changes in bowel habits that may have occurred decades earlier. For the physician, it is helpful when a patient identifies a time that their bowels changed from one pattern to another. This change may have involved a change in the bowel's consistency, frequency, or difficulty/ease of passage.

This change may or may not be associated with a traumatic event. Obviously, this is information more readily extractable if the change is of recent onset as opposed to a change that occurred decades prior. Further complicating matters is that these changes may progress slowly and ultimately develop a characteristic pattern that is typical for that individual. While no two people with IBS display the same symptoms, for a specific individual, symptoms ultimately become somewhat predictable.

Related to altered bowel habits are altered bowel transit and motility. Bowel transit relates to the time it takes for material to move through the bowel. Bowel motility describes the way the bowel contracts, such as in peristalsis. Bowel transit times and motility vary widely between individuals with and without IBS. People without IBS have, on average, six to eight "high-amplitude" peristaltic contractions daily, especially during meals and bowel movements. These normal contractions are significantly reduced in people with constipation-predominant IBS. Another type of altered gut motility is found in people with IBS who are fasting. These individuals can lose a basic type of small bowel peristaltic activity called the migrating motor complex. We also know that in IBS there are abnormal bowel contractions that can cause pain. Food can trigger altered bowel motility in people with IBS as can mental and physical stress, findings observed since the 1940s.

In general, there is a poor correlation between gut motility and IBS symptoms. Nevertheless, many experts believe that abnormal motility in the small and large intestines is responsible for the diarrhea, constipation, and abdominal pain characteristic of IBS.

BOWEL HYPERSENSITIVITY

People with IBS have significantly lower thresholds for bowel pain, and visceral or bowel hypersensitivity is common in IBS. Studies have found that it takes less mechanical bowel distention to create abdominal pain in people with IBS than it would take in those without IBS. This lower threshold for bowel pain is present in approximately two-thirds of people with IBS.

Various theories have been offered to explain visceral hypersensitivity and range from dysfunctional nerve endings to abnormalities in how the spinal cord and brain process information. Interactions between the gut and central nervous system are an area of intense research. Magnetic resonance imaging (MRI) and tomography scans show differences in discreet brain areas when comparing people with and without IBS. This research has helped us understand that the decreased pain thresholds and increased pain sensations so common with IBS may be related to how the brain processes information from the intestines as well as how the bowel interprets information from the brain.

ABDOMINAL PAIN

As far as physicians are concerned, if you don't have abdominal pain, you don't have IBS. Abdominal pain is perhaps the most disturbing and debilitating symptom of IBS. The pain can range from mild to moderate to severe and typically waxes and wanes, often being completely or partially relieved by defecation. This relief, however, is often only temporary, and the pain frequently recurs. Bloating may accompany the pain in some cases.

Sometimes abdominal pain is caused by a meal, a pattern that typically gets better with stool passage. Food-related IBS abdominal pain can be caused by a food allergy/intolerance or the fat/fiber content of the food. Pain typically occurs only during waking hours and rarely during sleep. In fact, abdominal pain that wakes an individual from sleep is usually associated with a more serious disorder and not caused by IBS.

IBS pain is often perceived as a dull, vague, cramplike sensation that does not localize to any particular part of the abdomen. Others describe a sharp or knifelike pain that can be referred to a specific area. Many people with IBS will experience both sensations together, with a sharp stabbing pain superimposed over an area of dull, nonlocalized pain. It is not uncommon for people with IBS to complain of having pain in multiple abdominal sites.

The pain can occur anywhere in the abdomen; however, the lower abdomen is most commonly affected, with the lower left abdomen particularly involved. This is why some people with IBS are misdiagnosed as having diverticular disease, as the symptoms of diverticulitis classically occur in the same area. Abdominal pain may radiate to the lower back, but this is uncommon in IBS.

Some people complain of pain in the upper left abdomen, or quadrant, which may actually be felt in the chest. IBS-related chest pain can be confused with heart pain, especially in people who have a diagnosis of heart disease. Pain that is localized to the upper left quadrant and caused by gas is known as the "splenic flexure syndrome." The splenic flexure is the part of the colon located near the spleen, and gas tends to accumulate there as it sits high in the abdomen.

Finally, people with IBS can also experience rectal pain that can range from mild to excruciating. Rectal pain is usually not localized and may be associated with the passage of small quantities of stool.

While we are not entirely certain what causes this pain, many experts suspect that bowel distention is responsible. The lower pain thresholds found in IBS may contribute to the frequency and severity of symptoms. This visceral hypersensitivity results from alterations in stretch receptors or spinal pathways for pain. Stretch receptors are part of the ENS and monitor bowel distention. It is suspected that in IBS, these stretch receptors may not be working normally and are sending signals to the brain that are interpreted as painful. The spinal cord receives information from the ENS and these ENS–spinal cord pathways may also be abnormal in some people with IBS. Further reflecting the dysfunctional perception of what may be normal physiological events are studies demonstrating that some people with IBS complain of increased symptoms from only mild distention of the gut.

These altered pathways, however, are not confined to the gut and spinal cord. PET scanning has demonstrated that, in people with IBS, different areas of the brain are activated by painful bowel stimuli when compared with people who do not have IBS. It has been suggested that decreased bowel transit times may play a role in IBS-related pain.

Other experts suspect that psychological factors predominate in IBS-related visceral hypersensitivity. Researchers examined the impact of psychological traits on altered pain sensitivity and concluded that somatization correlates significantly with pain thresholds. Somatization is a tendency to notice many bodily sensations and to interpret them as symptoms of disease.

Arguing against the role of emotions in gut hypersensitivity are studies that examine the reaction of IBS patients to skin pain. Somatization and anxiety are intimately related, and people who are anxious frequently display pain hypersensitivity in multiple organ systems. One review article examined several studies evaluating skin pain sensitivity in IBS and found that "patients with IBS [were] either similar to or less sensitive than healthy controls to painful stimulation of the skin." The authors concluded that "increased pain sensitivity is specific to the gastrointestinal tract [and] demonstrate that general psychological traits such as anxiety cannot explain lower threshold to distention-related pain." These authors, however, caution that the studies do not exclude the possibility that psychological traits change pain perceptions in the bowel.

Yet, we cannot deny the fact that, even in people without IBS, the bowel is often sensitive to emotional factors. These emotionally induced responses are described in both the small and large intestines. As you will learn in Chapter 4, the mind-bowel relationship has been extensively studied and documented. One author noted that "in studies of the large bowel, it has been observed that in those who perceive themselves as threatened in a given way, quantities of blood engorge the mucous membranes, and motility and secretion are augmented. It should also be recalled that every school boy is aware of the sensitivity of the colon as an organ for spontaneous emotional response."

Many researchers suspect that the bowel can be conditioned like a Pavlovian-conditioned reflex, so that for some people, IBS is a learned response to stress. It is no secret that overactivity of the bowel is a common reaction to anxiety, and the intestines can become "sensitized" in a susceptible individual. Indeed, most of us are familiar with "butterflies in the stomach" and other emotionally induced reactions such as stress-related diarrhea. This is why alternative therapies, like hypnotherapy, that utilize bowel "desensitization" often help people with IBS. Alternative therapies will be explored in more detail in Chapter 7.

It is clear that many factors are involved in IBS hypersensitivity. Both psychological and physical/organic factors play important roles in IBS-related visceral hypersensitivity, but the contribution of each varies from individual to individual. While multiple studies have documented the role physical factors play in gut hypersensitivity, a substantial body of literature indicates that psychological factors also make a significant contribution. In fact, researchers have known for years that the perception of pain is influenced by stress, relaxation, attention, and distraction. These mind-bowel interactions will be explored in more detail in Chapter 4.

GAS AND BLOATING

Everybody has gas, but people differ in the type and quantity of gas produced. This gas makes its presence known in multiple ways and can manifest as belching (burping) or as flatus (gas that is passed from the anus). Gas comes from several possible sources. Diet primarily determines how much gas we have, and personal experience will tell us which foods give us more gas.

Another major source of gas comes from bacteria that normally inhabit our bowels. Everybody has their own unique flora or bacteria in their gut, and variations and changes in normal gut flora can occur. There is evidence that people with IBS have abnormal gut "fermentation," often causing gas, due to dysfunctional gut flora.

What is a normal amount of gas? A reasonable amount would be that most people, on average, pass gas ten to fifteen times daily. While the number of gas passage events is fairly consistent among most people, the volume can vary significantly, from 476 to 1491 milliliters in a twenty-four-hour period. Much of what we call "gas" is actually air that we swallow while eating. (If you're concerned about how much gas you're making, try taking smaller bites of food and chewing with your mouth closed.)

The quantity of bowel gas also depends on how much is absorbed by the blood. A certain percentage of bowel gas is absorbed in the blood, and the amount absorbed can be influenced by bowel transit time. For example, the rapid bowel transit found in many people with IBS decreases the time blood has to absorb gas, leaving more gas in the bowel. This may explain why people with diarrhea-predominant IBS have increased gas. One British study speculated that rapid transit time in the small intestine might be associated with bloating; however, rapid small-bowel transit time is not universal in people with IBS. Nevertheless, it is suspected that this rapid delivery of food to the large intestine may result in "excessive fermentation," which leads to increased gas production.

Another source of bowel gas comes from swallowing air. Known as aerophagia, this mechanism appears to play a more significant role in people with anxiety, who tend to swallow more air.

Bowel Transit Time

One of the most helpful concepts in understanding IBS is bowel transit time—how long it takes for bowel contents to move through the small and large intestines. The average transit time for the ascending and transverse colon is fifteen hours, whereas the average transit time for the descending colon is three hours. If bowel contents move too fast and do not permit adequate time for nutrients and water to be absorbed, diarrhea may result. If bowel transit time is too slow, the stool becomes dehydrated, making it difficult to pass and resulting in constipation.

Transit time depends on multiple factors, including age, physical activity, medical conditions, diet, and drug use. Disease states can also affect bowel transit time: Bacterial or viral infections often cause diarrhea, whereas neurological conditions like Hirschsprung's disease can cause severe constipation. Hirschsprung's disease is a congenital disorder in which nerves are missing from the terminal colon and rectum, causing severe constipation as a result.

Marked variations in bowel transit time are seen in IBS, and some experts suspect that these variations may be responsible for the variable degrees of bowel dysfunction seen in the syndrome. Some studies have found that especially in IBS characterized by abdominal pain and bloating, there is rapid small bowel transit with a reduced colonic response to the food residue. But one group of researchers found that small bowel transit times were increased rather than decreased in pain/bloating-predominant IBS. This is opposite to what the previous group found. And people with diarrhea-predominant IBS report delayed small bowel transit times. Obviously, there is much we don't understand regarding correlating bowel transit time to IBS symptoms. However, deranged bowel motility does exist in IBS and more than likely plays a role in its symptoms.

Studies have shown that some people with IBS who complain of excessive gas actually have normal amounts of gas, a finding that may be related to altered interpretation of bowel sensory input. Driving home the fact that few, if any, generalizations can be made regarding IBS, we also know that some people with complaints of gas actually do have increased gas. In the final analysis, the documentation of gas in a person with IBS must be highly individualized, as some people with this complaint will have excess gas, and others will not.

A little-known fact for anyone who suffers from gas-related pain in the upper left quadrant of the abdomen or anterior chest is that this pain can occur from gas collecting in the splenic flexure. The splenic flexure is anatomically the highest part of the bowel when an individual is positioned upright and the area where gas rises and collects. Gas-induced colonic distention is implicated as one of the causes of IBS abdominal pain, particularly in splenic flexure syndrome. One trick to relieve this type of gas is to lie flat on your back and raise your buttocks so that your butt is higher than your abdomen. This way the gas rises naturally, traveling from your bowel to your rectum, where it can be passed.

While gas can certainly cause pain in the anterior chest, do not forget about the heart. Do not assume that anterior chest pain is caused by gas; it could also be caused by stomach acid or heart disease. If you have any chest pain, tell your doctor. This is especially true if you are over age fifty, have a history of or risk factors for heart disease, or your chest pain is accompanied by shortness of breath or sweating. In fact, if you have chest pain along with shortness of breath or sweating, you should call 911 or go to the nearest emergency room.

People with IBS also often suffer from bloating or the perception of bloating. Bloating is a little more complicated because the subjective sensation of feeling bloated can be markedly different from being objectively bloated. Subjectively, bloating refers to feeling "full," while objective measurements of bloating require an increase in abdominal girth. But some people with IBS who complain of being bloated are found not to be bloated at all. Conversely, there are people with IBS who complain of being bloated and are actually objectively bloated. When objectively bloated, IBS sufferers relate their symptoms to the lower abdomen. In IBS, bloating symptoms are usually mild or nonexistent in the morning and progressively get worse throughout the day.

While increased gas probably plays a large role in the bloating in people with IBS, other factors make a contribution. Nevertheless, people with IBS do have a tendency to be gassy and bloated due primarily to dysfunctional rapid bowel transport and increased colonic gas production.

In addition to gas and bloating, many people with IBS complain of passing small amounts of stool with increased amounts of whitish or clear mucus. Mucus is normally found in the bowel and helps stool to pass. Despite extensive investigations, why people with IBS have increased bowel mucus remains a mystery.

CONSTIPATION

Constipation is one of the most common medical complaints, and, along with diarrhea, accounts for approximately 50 percent of all specialist referrals. It is estimated that 3 to 17 percent of the United States population suffers from chronic constipation; however, the actual number is probably closer to 3 percent when strict criteria for defining constipation are used. The severity of constipation can range from a mild nuisance to a potentially life-threatening disorder and may be related to many syndromes and diseases, from IBS to colorectal cancer. Most people with constipation-predominant IBS have constipation for several days or weeks, with the pattern occasionally interrupted by a bout of diarrhea.

Constipation is difficult to define, and many experts disagree over its meaning. This is complicated by the fact that ideas regarding normal bowel habits vary widely from person to person and are shaped by our parents, society, and the popular media. As a young physician, I became convinced that the entire world was constipated since I heard this complaint over and over again. When I did research and my understanding of normal bowel function matured, I realized that true constipation is rare.

According to the textbook definition, constipation can be defined as having fewer than three stools per week. Many people are surprised to learn that the number of stools per day or week is only part of the constipation equation. Also included in the evaluation are complaints of difficult-to-pass stools, abnormal straining or time to pass stool, a sensation of incomplete evacuation, and complaints of abdominal "fullness" and "hard" stools. Also helpful in establishing a diagnosis of constipation is a history of using enemas or manual disimpaction. But even this history is not totally reliable, since some people regularly use enemas or laxatives when they are not needed.

Constipation can be either acute or chronic, with acute constipation usually raising the most concern, as it may indicate a more serious condition. Most cases of constipation are caused by inadequate fiber intake. There are, however, multiple medications and medical conditions that can also cause constipation, and it is important for the physician to rule these out prior to making a diagnosis of IBS. Medications are another common cause of constipation, particularly calcium channel-blockers used to treat heart conditions and antidepressants, agents that ironically are also frequently used to treat IBS.

Perhaps the most important underlying medical condition to rule out is cancer. This is especially true after age fifty, as colon cancer can cause constipation or diarrhea. Bowel obstruction is another dangerous cause of constipation that can be related to cancer, a stricture, inadequate blood supply, or an inflammatory process. Sometimes people who are constipat-

Warning Sign:
A Change in Bowel Habits

In my practice, I see many people who say they are constipated; however, after further examination, I often find that their bowel habits are actually normal. Many people carry some emotional baggage when it comes to their bowels. Beliefs regarding what is a "normal" bowel habit are in large part shaped by our parents and the media. So, let's set the record straight.

Some people believe that they must move their bowels once daily to be healthy. Nothing can be further from the truth. Bowel habits, like people, vary widely, and what is normal for me may not be normal for you. Some people have two bowel movements a day, others have only one bowel movement every two days. Both of these patterns can be perfectly normal as long as they do not represent a significant change from previous bowel behavior.

This is a key warning sign for all gastrointestinal disorders: a *change* in bowel habits. If you have been having a bowel movement once every two days for the past thirty years, chances are this is just how your body works, and you are not constipated. Conversely, if you have been having a bowel movement every three days for many years and now you are going twice a day, something may be wrong. When evaluating bowel disorders, physicians look for many things, but one of the most important symptoms is a *change* in bowel habits.

ed have a normal colon, and it's the anus that is affected, such as in cases of painful, large hemorrhoids or anal fissures.

People with nervous system problems like multiple sclerosis, Parkinson's disease, and any type of spinal cord injury are frequently constipated. So too are people with hypothyroidism, one of the most common glandular conditions in America. Mechanical disorders that involve the colon can cause constipation, including rectal prolapse and disorders of the muscles that control the anus and pelvic floor.

Megacolon, an abnormal dilatation of the descending colon, can also cause constipation and is an occasional complication of laxative abuse. People with depression and eating disorders can also find themselves constipated. Another cause of chronic constipation is called "idiopathic constipation," involving unusually slow transit time through the bowel, especially the ascending and transverse colon, with a decreased number of colonic contractions. And, as many women can tell you, you can be perfectly healthy and still be constipated if you are pregnant. Finally, being a couch potato may be hazardous to your bowel—people who are physically inactive, or who become immobilized secondary to a medical condition like a stroke, often become constipated.

As you can see, there are many causes of chronic constipation, and only after these and numerous other conditions have been excluded can a physician make a diagnosis of IBS. For more than 90 percent of people, there will be no identifiable cause for their constipation, and most of these individuals will respond to increased exercise coupled with adequate fluid and fiber intake.

Evaluating and Treating Constipation

In addition to performing a complete history and physical exam, your doctor will be especially interested in whether or not your constipation is of recent onset. In general, new constipation is of more concern than constipation that has existed for decades. Your doctor will also be interested in the prescription and over-the-counter medications you are taking, as certain medications are notorious for causing constipation.

Your doctor will also perform a rectal exam. While we will discuss diagnostic tests in Chapter 3, let me emphasize that the rectal exam is an extremely important and easy test that aids in the diagnosis of a variety of medical conditions, ranging from colon cancer to increased anal sphincter tone. Your doctor will also test your blood for electrolyte disorders and anemia, both of which may be caused by a variety of gastrointestinal disorders. Also expect to have your thyroid-stimulating hormone tested, since hypothyroidism can cause constipation.

Depending on what is discovered, you may walk away from your doctor's office with some fiber or with orders for additional tests. Most doctors agree that symptoms suggestive of a more serious disease, like anemia, weight loss, and rectal bleeding, demand aggressive investigation. If you have any of these symptoms, expect to receive a colonoscopy or a sigmoidoscopy with barium enema. (To learn more about these tests, see Chapter 3.) Other diagnostic procedures may be indicated depending on what your doctor finds.

Approximately 95 percent of patients with simple constipation respond to the treatment measures described below. The remaining 5 percent are considered to have "intractable" constipation and demand further evaluation that may include evaluation of bowel transit time and measurement of pelvic and rectal muscle function. In this group of "intractable" individuals, a readily identifiable cause for constipation can be found in only about 30 percent.

Most cases of uncomplicated constipation have an excellent response to regular exercise, increased water intake, and fiber supplementation. Your healthcare provider will also want you to develop good bowel habits. The bowel, much like a house pet, is trainable, and the passage of stool is both a reflexive and a learned response. Most people feel the urge to defecate after breakfast, and it is suggested that you spend no more than twenty minutes on the toilet after breakfast. While in the bathroom, do not strain excessively, and if you do not move your bowel after twenty minutes, leave the bathroom and return only when you feel the need.

Depending on your symptoms and findings, you may be prescribed a laxative or an enema; however, for most healthcare practitioners, these are the treatments of last resort. If bowel transit time is slow, most physicians will attempt a trial of a bulking agent like psyllium. Rarely, laxatives like milk of magnesia or lactulose will be used to encourage bowel movements. Enemas and laxatives should only be used under the supervision of a healthcare provider. Even though these products are available over the counter, you should not take it upon yourself to use laxatives or enemas. Most people with constipation respond well to the simple measures described above. If you are one of those who has constipation that is recalcitrant to conservative therapy, you will probably be referred to a specialist, such as a gastroenterologist.

Surgical intervention is usually reserved for those who have anatomic defects or have documented slow-transit constipation but fail to respond to aggressive medical therapy. Those with a diagnosis of megacolon or megarectum are also considered surgical candidates. Surgery is used in only a small minority of patients as most cases respond to basic interventions. For people with anal sphincter spasm or pelvic muscle dysfunction, biofeedback with muscle relaxation is often successfully employed, a topic covered in more detail in Chapter 7.

Constipation in IBS

People with constipation-predominant IBS typically experience several days or weeks of constipation that is ultimately interrupted by diarrhea. This alternating pattern is one of the most important defining features of IBS. In IBS, constipation usually begins in childhood to early adulthood as an infrequent complaint that progressively becomes more common, ultimately establishing itself as constipation-predominant IBS. Because there is a history of chronic constipation that may have existed for decades, some people have a history of enema or laxative use. Unfortunately, people with IBS should avoid enemas and laxatives because these products can make symptoms worse and result in potentially dangerous complications.

One of the first things I do when evaluating an individual for bowel

---

What Is a Normal Stool?

What does a normal stool look like? You're probably chuckling to yourself because you can't believe I'm writing about this; however, this is an important question. Let's face it, conversation about stools does not typically occur during cocktail parties, and most of us only know what our stools look like. Like the definitions of constipation and diarrhea, what a "normal" stool looks like depends on the individual. A normal stool is determined by several factors, especially what you eat and the medications you take. Stool morphology is also influenced by how fast your bowel moves: The slower your bowel moves, the harder the stool. For example, slow bowel transit is normally associated with hard, pelletlike stools that are more difficult to pass than large, slightly softer stools. Conversely, rapid bowel transit usually produces a watery, loose stool. A "normal" stool can best be described as one that is neither too hard nor too soft and is easy to pass.

dysfunction is to remove all unnecessary medications and see how their bowels behave when not influenced by pharmaceuticals, enemas, or laxatives. Most people with normal bowel function can experience occasional bouts of constipation, and some may attempt to self-medicate with a laxative or enema. As I will emphasize throughout this book, the bowel is a trainable organ, and abuse of these products can make the bowel dependent on their use to function. Once the bowel becomes dependent on laxatives or enemas, the stage is set for a vicious cycle of constipation followed by laxative or enema abuse. Ultimately, the bowel becomes unresponsive to laxatives and enemas, and this results in more serious complications. If you happen to be using enemas or laxatives, I strongly suggest that, under the supervision of a healthcare professional, you discontinue these products and see what happens. Some of you may be surprised to learn that you don't have IBS, and your problem actually lies in your pattern of laxative or enema use.

While people with IBS can pass many different stool types, the typical constipated stool is hard because it is dehydrated. Some people with IBS characterized by colonic or rectal spasms may complain of thin stools, often described as "ribbon-like" or "pencil-like." Thin stools, especially stools that were once "normal" in caliber and progressively became thin, can also indicate a more serious problem like colon cancer and should always be investigated by a physician. Others with IBS may complain of "marble-like," small, hard stools, otherwise known as scybalous.

Complaints of straining, difficulty, or pain in stool passage are also common in constipation-predominant IBS. When pain is associated with constipation, the typical pattern is one of increasing pain with increasing constipation. While this pain may be relieved by defecation, many people feel that they did not completely empty their bowels once defecation was achieved; this often leads to excessive time in the bathroom spent attempting to "fully" empty their bowel.

DIARRHEA

One billion people are afflicted annually by diarrhea worldwide. While diarrhea is an occasional albeit uncomfortable complaint for the majority of people, for the individual with IBS diarrhea can be a debilitating daily ordeal. In the United States, approximately 100 million people are stricken annually, and it is estimated that diarrhea results in 250,000 hospitalizations and 3,000 deaths yearly.

Diarrhea can be a mere nuisance, or it can evolve into a life-threatening disorder. Like constipation, diarrhea can be associated with multiple disorders, ranging from IBS to hyperthyroidism to colorectal cancer. Further challenging physicians, the clinical severity of diarrhea often does not match the severity of the causative disorder. In other words, mild diarrhea may be associated with a potentially deadly cancer, whereas debilitating severe diarrhea can be found in some people with IBS, which is not life-threatening but may be debilitating.

The definition of diarrhea is controversial and even today remains nebulous at best. According to standard textbooks, diarrhea is defined as passage of abnormally liquid (or unformed) stools at an increased frequency. Another way to define diarrhea is the passage of more than three stools a day. This, however, does not paint an entirely accurate picture, as the definition of diarrhea must consider both the stool number and consistency. Equally important is how the bowel habits have changed—for diarrhea, this specifically means an increase in the number of daily bowel movements. Hence, diarrhea can be characterized by an increase in frequency and/or volume of stool. Duration of diarrhea is another important consideration. Acute diarrhea is defined as lasting for less than two weeks, whereas chronic diarrhea lasts over four weeks. Persistent diarrhea lies somewhere between these acute and chronic states, lasting two to four weeks.

The most common cause of diarrhea worldwide is viral or bacterial. Other causes of diarrhea include fecal incontinence, the inability to control passage of fecal material, which usually results from an anatomic abnormality or a nervous system disorder. Inflammation of the bowel can also cause diarrhea and is seen in conditions like Crohn's disease and ulcerative colitis, which often produce bloody diarrhea. Proctitis, a type of rectal inflammation, can cause diarrhea with rectal pain.

For people with IBS, the evaluation of acute diarrhea becomes relevant only during an acute exacerbation. Since IBS has periods of exacerbation and remission, an exacerbation may represent the natural IBS course or another cause of acute diarrhea superimposed on IBS. During an IBS exacerbation, infectious and other causes of acute diarrhea should always be considered. If you have IBS and have a sudden increase in diarrhea accompanied by fever, chills, or vomiting, you should notify your doctor, as these symptoms are more indicative of infection. If you have the misfortune of experiencing infection-related diarrhea, the overwhelming majority of infections resolve in several days with no permanent ill effects. The most important thing anyone can do when stricken with acute diarrhea is drink plenty of fluids. In fact, it is dehydration that lands most people in the hospital rather than the infection itself.

As mentioned previously, medications are another cause of diarrhea. In most cases of medication-induced diarrhea, symptoms occur in close proximity to starting the new medicine. Hence, the cause is usually rapidly recognized by the patient or their physician, and the offending medication is discontinued. Nevertheless, it is important that you and your doctor carefully review all the prescription and nonprescription medications you are taking. The number of medications that can cause diarrhea is extensive, including antibiotics, antidepressants, antacids, asthma drugs, cancer chemotherapy, heart medications, high blood pressure agents, nonsteroidal anti-inflammatory drugs (NSAIDs), and laxatives.

Evaluating and Treating Acute Diarrhea

One of the challenges in evaluating diarrhea is to distinguish acute diarrhea from chronic diarrhea. This is especially true in conditions like lactose intolerance and inflammatory bowel disease, where an acute bout of diarrhea may actually be the harbinger of a more chronic process. Like the evaluation of constipation, expect to have a complete history and physical exam that may include blood work and diagnostic tests.

Since most episodes of acute diarrhea resolve quickly, most physicians will adopt a "wait and see" approach for the first bout of acute diarrhea, only offering reassurance and advice to stay well hydrated. Of all the symptoms associated with acute diarrhea, it is usually dehydration that causes the most trouble. In fact, dehydration is one of the leading causes of death from diarrhea worldwide. If you have an acute episode of diarrhea, no matter what the cause, it is critical that you stay well hydrated.

For most cases of acute diarrhea, this is appropriate, and further diagnostic tests with more aggressive treatment is not indicated. In fact, the vast majority of acute diarrhea cases are best left to follow their natural course. Treatment with antibiotics is generally taboo, since the antibiotics can potentially cause more problems than they solve. Symptoms that demand further investigation include severe abdominal pain, fever, bloody diarrhea, dehydration, symptoms that last more than two days without improving, age over seventy, and a history of being immunocompromised. For these patients, a more aggressive workup is indicated that may consist of a stool sample, a sigmoidoscopy or colonoscopy, or an abdominal X-ray or CAT scan.

Doctors rarely prescribe antimotility agents to control diarrhea, usually employed only in those cases of diarrhea that are not accompanied by fever or blood. For infectious diarrhea, the rapid transit of bowel contents that causes the symptom we call "diarrhea" is actually a defense mechanism that rapidly rids the bowel of the offending organism. By giving an antimotility agent, you run the risk of keeping the organism in the bowel for a longer period of time, thereby giving it additional opportunity to cause trouble. An alternative to antimotility agents that works for diarrhea is bismuth subsalicylate, found in over-the-counter preparations like Pepto-Bismol, for which the same cautions apply.

While antibiotics are generally avoided in acute diarrhea, they are clearly indicated in certain cases. Whether or not you are prescribed antibiotics depends on symptom severity, laboratory results, and your other medical problems. While the list of organisms that can cause infectious diarrhea is extensive, one organism people with IBS should know about is *Giardia.* The organism is usually transmitted by drinking water that has been contaminated by human or animal feces. Known for causing explosive, foul-smelling diarrhea, giardiasis classically causes chronic diarrhea. The bug especially afflicts travelers and campers, but if you're being evaluated for IBS, make sure you are specifically tested for this organism.

Chronic Diarrhea

Unlike acute diarrhea, most cases of chronic diarrhea are functional or inflammatory. One of the more common mechanisms of chronic diarrhea is a disorder that involves the transport of electrolytes and fluids in the bowel. Known as "secretory" diarrhea, the classic symptom is profuse, painless, and watery diarrhea. Alcohol and laxative use are common causes. This is one of the reasons why people with IBS should avoid alcohol, as it can damage the bowel's lining, resulting in abnormal transport of water and electrolytes. Medications are another major cause of secretory diarrhea. This is why you and your doctor need to carefully review all prescription and nonprescription medications, since identification of an offending medication can save you significant trouble. Secretory diarrhea can also occur following bowel surgery or in any disease that interferes with the colon's ability to manage fluids and electrolytes, such as carcinoid tumor, gastrinoma, and thyroid cancer.

"Osmotic" diarrhea is caused by the bowel's inability to digest a specific substance, such as a laxative. This indigestible product is retained in the intestine, where it draws excess water into the bowel through an osmotic effect. Perhaps the most common example of osmotic diarrhea is lactose intolerance, a condition characterized by the inability to digest the sugar found in dairy products. Lactose intolerance is estimated to afflict 30 percent of the United States population and is often confused with IBS. (To learn more about lactose intolerance, see Chapter 5.)

While most diarrheas are accompanied by rapid bowel transit, disorders of gut motility can also cause chronic diarrhea. Two of the most common conditions in this category are hyperthyroidism and diabetes, both of which can cause alterations in gut motility that result in diarrhea. Also included in this category is IBS, which is characterized by dysfunctional bowel motor activity.

Malabsorption syndromes, particularly fat malabsorption, can also cause chronic diarrhea. These syndromes are typically associated with pancreatic or liver disease or from long-standing alcohol abuse. What often distinguishes these disorders from IBS is the nature of the diarrhea and the accompanying weight loss. Other causes of malabsorption include celiac sprue and Whipple's disease. People with celiac sprue cannot digest gluten, an insoluble protein found in wheat and grains. Whipple's disease is caused by the bacteria *Tropheryma whippelii,* which can infect multiple organs including the bowel, resulting in diarrhea and weight loss.

One of the most important causes of chronic diarrhea is inflammatory bowel disease (IBD), specifically Crohn's disease and ulcerative colitis, conditions that typically provoke bloody diarrhea. The severity of IBD ranges from mild to severe, and the symptoms can mimic IBS. While bloody diarrhea is classic for IBD, this disease can also be present without bloody diarrhea. Also distinguishing IBD from IBS is that IBD is potentially life-threatening; hence, this disease must be considered by your physician. The good news is that IBD can be managed with medication and that superior treatments are being actively investigated.

Diagnosing Chronic Diarrhea

The workup of chronic diarrhea tends to be more intensive and invasive than acute diarrhea. Standard to this workup is a complete history and a physical with blood tests and a stool sample. Most physicians will have a clinical suspicion regarding what is causing chronic diarrhea and in the absence of obvious "warning signs" will initiate treatment prior to undergoing an extensive workup. For instance, if you noticed that your diarrhea began shortly after taking a new medication, your doctor will probably stop that medication prior to an extensive evaluation. For those individuals who do not respond to initial measures, a more extensive workup is indicated, which can include repeated stool collection, abdominal imaging, sigmoidoscopy, or full colonoscopy. While the large bowel is of primary concern, some patients may need their stomach, small bowel, or other parts of their body examined.

Diarrhea and IBS

Diarrhea is a common complaint in IBS, and several types of diarrhea are typical. One form is called pseudodiarrhea and is characterized by the frequent passing of small quantities of stool. This type of diarrhea carries the prefix "pseudo" because the weight of the stool is usually less than 200 grams daily. Besides having small, frequent bowel movements, people with pseudodiarrhea often have fecal urgency, a strong, sudden urge to defecate. While IBS-associated diarrhea varies from person to person, it typically consists of small quantities of loose stool that are often passed in the morning and after a meal. Tenesmus can also occur and is characterized by a painful spasm of the anal sphincter with an urgent need to defecate.

While the bowel habits of individuals with IBS vary widely, the following pattern is prototypical. Many people with IBS will have a normally formed stool in the morning. Shortly after passing this stool, however, a softer, less formed stool is passed. As the day progresses, any subsequently passed stool will be looser and looser. Associated with these stools is abdominal pain that is usually completely or partially relieved by defecation. This abdominal pain usually recurs later in the day.

Postprandial diarrhea, which is diarrhea that occurs after a meal, is also seen in IBS. What typically happens is that shortly after eating breakfast, lunch, or dinner, the individual will experience an urgent need to pass stool that may or may not be accompanied by pain. Postprandial diarrhea is often accompanied by large quantities of gas and fluid, which, as any sufferer will tell you, leads to an explosive mixture. As a rule, the more food consumed, the greater the risk of postprandial diarrhea.

Diarrhea Survival Guide

One of the most important things you can do while having diarrhea is to make sure you get enough calories and stay hydrated. In fact, the most dangerous thing about diarrhea is dehydration and electrolyte derangements. Water and orange juice take care of the hydration and potassium, and most salted foods help to replace your sodium. There are also several rehydration formulas available, including Pedialyte, Ceralyte, and Infalyte. Stay in close contact with your healthcare professional, who can individualize treatment based on your symptoms and medical history. This is especially true for people with diabetes, who can experience dangerously low or high blood sugar levels during bouts of diarrhea.

If you have chronic diarrhea, have your potassium level checked periodically. While potassium supplements are available, they are potentially dangerous and should only be used under the supervision of a physician. If you are concerned about potassium, I suggest orange juice or a daily banana, both rich in potassium. As for sodium or salt, given the typical American diet, sodium is rarely a problem for the vast majority of people with diarrhea. Sodium supplements are occasionally used in heavily perspiring athletes; however, most people don't need them, and they should only be used under a doctor's supervision.

Chapter 3

Diagnosing IBS

A s mentioned previously, determining if someone has irritable bowel is a diagnosis of exclusion. But what do we mean by this? A diagnosis of IBS can only be made once other diseases have been ruled out. In other words, before physicians can definitively diagnose IBS, they must be sure that conditions such as lactose intolerance, gastroesophageal reflux disease, peptic ulcer disease, and colon cancer have been eliminated as possibilities. This is because the symptoms found in IBS are also displayed by multiple gastrointestinal disorders.

The evaluation of IBS must take into consideration the totality of the patient: the physical exam, medical history, and laboratory/radiographic results. The most critical information comes not from diagnostic testing but from what you tell your doctor. Without question, an IBS diagnosis often rests on your medical history, with diagnostic tests only serving to rule out other conditions.

QUESTIONS YOU NEED TO ASK YOURSELF

"Know thyself"—those words ring true for every part of life, but they are especially pertinent for people with IBS, because the more you know about IBS the better you can control it. Learning about IBS and knowing what type of IBS you have will enable you to live a healthy life. Equally important, asking yourself questions about your IBS will give you important information to help you and your healthcare provider develop a successful treatment plan.

What triggers your IBS? Without a doubt, this is the most important question. Most people with IBS can identify several things they know will irritate their bowels. Finding these triggers and eliminating them from your life may set you free. I hope that, after reading this book, many of you will find that magic trigger and rid yourself of IBS. Most of you, however, will have to do some detective work. There will be some trial and error, but if you are patient and methodical, you will discover what causes your IBS.

You probably know a lot about your IBS already, and most of you can name five things that aggravate your symptoms. The most important task is to ask five basic questions each time you have an attack:

- What am I doing?

- What are my symptoms?

- What was the last meal I had?

- Do I know what set off this attack?

- How severe is this attack?

To answer these questions, you'll need to start an "IBS diary," a journal to track your answers to these questions, along with the date and time of the attack. Everyone has their own method of keeping an IBS diary, but the following headings are standard and will help you and your physician immensely in determining what upsets your bowels:

Date: Date attack started.

Time: Time you first noticed symptoms.

Location: Where you are at the beginning of the attack.

Circumstances: What you are doing when the attack started.

Foods Eaten: What was your last meal? Was it breakfast, lunch, or dinner? Record what you had and any snacks in between.

Trigger: What triggered the attack, if you know or suspect. If you only suspect, put a "?" next to the trigger.

Severity: How severe you believe the attack is; use a mild-moderate-severe scale.

Symptoms During Attack: How many bowel movements did you have in a twenty-four-hour period? How many days did you not have a bowel movement? What other symptoms were there? For instance, belching, nausea, bloating, or abdominal pain; rate the severity of each. Rate your abdominal pain on a scale of 0 to 10: 0 for no pain and 10 for the worst pain.

Treatment/Interventions: How did you abort the exacerbation? For example, what type and how much medicine you used or what you did in an attempt to relieve your symptoms. If you didn't do anything, write "nothing."

Time to Resolution: How soon after the intervention did the symptoms resolve?

Duration of Attack: How long did the exacerbation last, from the time you first noticed symptoms to the time the attack was over?

Keeping an IBS diary may seem like a lot of trouble, but it can help you and your healthcare professional find out what triggers your attacks and develop a plan for avoiding those triggers. Furthermore, you may be surprised that the simple act of keeping a diary may actually help your symptoms improve. I am hoping that by recording this data, you will begin to recognize patterns. For instance, you may find that your IBS tends to be worse after eating a particular food. I also want you to share your IBS diary with your physician and perhaps a trusted friend or two—a fresh eye may discover patterns that you can't see.

INTERROGATION TIME

It's time to ask some hard questions and discover what exacerbates your IBS. Before we begin, take a moment to write down five to ten things you know trigger your IBS symptoms. In answering these questions, we'll find that some IBS triggers are easy to identify and remove, whereas others may be more difficult to determine. The most important thing you can do right now is avoid known IBS triggers and stay true to your best friend, your IBS diary. What follows is a list of questions that, while far from exhaustive, offers an excellent start to get you thinking about your IBS and what sets it off.

When did your symptoms first start? One of the most important questions you need to ask is when you first noticed that something changed with respect to your bowel. As indicated earlier, most people with IBS first experience symptoms in adolescence or early adulthood. Depending on how long you've had your symptoms, some of you may only have to think back several years, whereas others will have several decades. The answer to this question, however, can yield important clues about the cause of your symptoms. Some people with IBS can relate the start of their symptoms to a traumatic life event. The answer to this simple but profound question can have a dramatic impact on how your IBS is managed.

How long have your symptoms lasted? This is related to the previous query, but sometimes asking the same question in a different way can help you remember.

What aggravates your symptoms? Knowing what irritates your bowels, then taking positive steps to avoid that trigger, can do more for you than any medicine or supplement.

What makes your symptoms better? While it is always preferable to avoid known triggers, the next best thing is to know what makes you feel better. In other words, of all the treatments for IBS, what works for you?

What does your stool normally look like? If you don't normally look at your stools, now is the time to start. Are your stools hard, soft, or watery? Does your stool come out as multiple little balls or in one large movement? What the stool looks like can give your healthcare provider important clues.

What is your symptom pattern? Do you have symptoms daily, weekly, or monthly? How long do your symptoms typically last—days, weeks, or months?

How many times daily do you have a bowel movement? The number will vary from person to person. This question is especially important for people with diarrhea.

How many times weekly do you have a bowel movement? Once, twice, never? This number is important for those with constipation.

Do you have fecal incontinence? Fecal incontinence, the inability to control fecal material from leaving the anus, can be caused by many problems besides IBS.

Do you have weight loss, fever, or bloody stools? These are warning signs that are not associated with IBS. If you have any of these symptoms, see your doctor immediately.

Have you ever traveled outside the United States, camped, or drunk water from a natural source like a stream, river, lake, or pond? The parasite *Giardia* can infect travelers and campers, producing chronic symptoms similar to IBS.

What medications are you taking? Medications may cause acute and chronic diarrhea or constipation, so it is important to rule these out as a cause of your symptoms.

Have you changed your diet? Food allergies and intolerances are common and can cause abdominal pain and diarrhea.

CLINICAL DIAGNOSIS OF IBS

Diagnosing IBS can be challenging because many of the symptoms associated with this syndrome are nonspecific and can be found in other gastrointestinal disorders. This is why some people who are ultimately diagnosed with IBS undergo an extensive medical workup.

Like the syndrome itself, the diagnosis of IBS and the tests necessary to establish the diagnosis have been the subject of controversy and only recently have been agreed upon and standardized. At the very minimum, most physicians will perform a complete history and physical exam with accompanying blood tests. However, other diagnostic tests are often needed, depending on the age of the patient. For most people under age fifty, this means a flexible sigmoidoscopy. For those over age fifty, a full colonoscopy or flexible sigmoidoscopy with barium enema is indicated.

While diagnostic studies are helpful to rule out serious diseases, most of these tests are normal in people with IBS. IBS is primarily a clinical diagnosis—that is, the symptoms are used to diagnose the syndrome, with ancillary tests employed to rule out other disorders that may mimic IBS. Most physicians use the International Working Team (Rome) Criteria to diagnose IBS. These Rome criteria have recently been modified to reflect the growing understanding of IBS. According to the new Rome II criteria, IBS is now defined as twelve weeks or more in the past year of abdominal discomfort or pain that has two of the following features:

1. Relieved with defecation

2. Onset associated with a change in frequency of stool

3. Onset associated with a change in consistency of stool

Additionally, the following are supportive symptoms of IBS, not diagnostic criteria, if present on at least 25 percent of occasions or days:

• Abnormal stool frequency (greater than three bowel movements per day or less than three per week)

• Abnormal stool form (lumpy/hard or loose/watery stool)

• Abnormal stool passage (straining, urgency, or feeling of incomplete evacuation)

• Passage of mucus

• Bloating or feeling of abdominal distention

While the Rome criteria are not perfect, they have helped physicians and patients think in a systematic way about IBS and are important in establishing a diagnosis.

DIFFERENTIAL DIAGNOSIS OF IBS

There are certain symptoms that are not normally seen in IBS, symptoms that set off alarms in the minds of physicians. For instance, symptoms that develop slowly are not usually seen in IBS. As the "bowel sleeps as we sleep," symptoms that wake a person from sleep are also not normally associated with IBS. Since IBS usually first manifests during adolescence or early adulthood, people who start having bowel complaints during old age are unlikely to have IBS. Also arguing against a diagnosis of IBS are rectal bleeding, weight loss, dehydration, and bloody or fatty stools—all point to other conditions. Finally, new symptoms that occur after having a history of relative "stability" typically argue against an IBS diagnosis.

Certain symptoms demand a more thorough and immediate investigation. Tell your doctor about these "alarm symptoms," and he or she should ask you about them as well. Alarm symptoms include anemia, bloody stools, blood from the rectum, weight loss, loss of appetite, fever, dehydration, severe diarrhea or constipation, fecal impaction, and a personal or family history of colon cancer, celiac sprue, or inflammatory bowel disease. Finally, symptoms suggestive of IBS that begin after age fifty also deserve a more extensive workup.

The term "differential diagnosis" essentially means the list of disorders a physician must consider in order to explain a particular set of complaints and/or findings. Many medical and nonmedical conditions can cause symptoms that may be confused with IBS and should be excluded by a physician prior to establishing a diagnosis. While the following list is far from complete, it offers a representative list of the conditions a physician should consider: anal fissure, anismus, bowel obstruction, cancer, Chagas' disease, depression, descending perineum syndrome, diverticular disease, eating disorders, endometriosis, hemorrhoids, Hirschsprung's disease, hypercalcemia, hypothyroidism, infection, inflammatory bowel disease, ischemia (inadequate blood supply), malabsorption, side effects from medications, megacolon, multiple sclerosis, Parkinson's disease, pelvic floor/musculature dysfunction, pregnancy complications, rectal prolapse, spinal cord injury, stricture, and systemic sclerosis.

TESTS FOR IBS

People are usually less anxious when they know what to expect. Be forewarned: When you visit a doctor for IBS, be prepared to be asked some very blunt questions. While some of these questions may seem intrusive and even "gross," they are vital and necessary to arrive at an accurate diagnosis. Once again, being asked these questions should not be viewed as an insult or offense. Doctors are in the job of finding out what is causing problems and fixing them. In fact, I would be more concerned about the physician who does not ask these questions. You should expect and demand that your doctor cover all the bases and assume nothing. Only by these honest questions and answers can a healthcare professional help you.

You will be asked about your complete medical and medication history. Medications are a common cause of gastrointestinal upset, and your doctor will be especially interested in what prescription and over-the-counter medications you take. Intense attention will also be directed at your diet, looking for food allergies or lactose intolerance. Don't be surprised if your doctor asks how you feel about yourself and your home life. These questions do not imply that your symptoms are in your head; rather, given the intricate and profound mind-body interactions that we all experience, such questions are normal and appropriate. Also, because of the association between IBS and physical/sexual abuse, be prepared to be asked about these issues.

You should expect your physician to consider the whole you, not just the medical you. Illness is more than just a physical complaint having dynamics that revolve around organ systems, environment, and personal life. Expect and demand that your doctor take the entirety of your existence into consideration. If he or she doesn't, perhaps you should find yourself another healthcare professional.

Besides a thorough medical and social history, you should expect to receive a complete physical exam. You may be surprised to learn that the vast majority of people with IBS have a normal physical exam; often there are no physical findings diagnostic of IBS. Expect that most doctors will give you a complete physical, paying attention to all organ systems; however, special attention will be devoted to poking and prodding the abdomen, as this is "where the money is" with respect to IBS. Blood tests will also be ordered to check for any abnormalities that may be related to your symptoms.

Finally, you can also expect a rectal exam. During the rectal exam, your doctor will insert a lubricated, gloved finger inside your rectum. You will feel some mild discomfort and pressure during the exam, a sensation similar to needing to have a bowel movement. Your doctor will insert a finger as far as possible inside your rectum in order to assess as much of the bowel as possible. This exam is important not only to detect abnormal growths but also to determine how tight your anus is. An anus that is either too tight or too loose can be caused by several medical conditions, including nerve problems. Abnormal anal tone can also result in constipation or diarrhea.

Your doctor will collect some stool during the rectal exam to test for blood. You may also be given stool sample cards to take home along with instructions on proper collection techniques. Visual and physical examination of the anus is also important because high anal sphincter tone, or a too tense anus, can cause constipation, whereas anal fissures or hemorrhoids can cause painful defecation. If you're a man, expect your doctor to check your prostate; if you're a woman, your doctor may perform a pelvic exam. Some gynecological disorders can cause abdominal pain in women and need to be excluded before a diagnosis of IBS can be made.

Most doctors end their examination with the rectal exam and follow up with recommendations that may be modified by blood test results. You can expect to see your doctor several times during the months following your initial visit. With time, however, and hopefully as your symptoms improve, these visits will become less frequent.

While medical practice varies from doctor to doctor, there are certain recommendations and tests that you can expect. Since lactose intolerance is common, most doctors will recommend that you eat a lactose-free diet for at least two weeks. This is especially true if you have bloating or evidence of increased gas. You can also expect to receive either a double contrast or single contrast barium enema, with or without a sigmoidoscopy or full colonoscopy. For those patients with diarrhea, a small bowel series may also be ordered. To learn more about these tests, see their individual sections below.

Sometimes, more extensive testing is needed. Most doctors agree that, in the absence of warning signs, the fewer tests the better. With respect to warning signs, of particular concern are complaints of rectal bleeding, bloody stools, fever, weight loss, and anemia. Any of these symptoms will prompt a physician to initiate a more aggressive evaluation to rule out serious diseases, such as cancer or inflammatory bowel disease. Your symptoms will ultimately dictate which tests your doctor orders. Finally, if you're over the age of fifty and never had a sigmoidoscopy or colonoscopy, your doctor will probably recommend that you receive one, as either of these tests are recommended as a standard screening exam after age fifty.

Blood Tests

Most people are familiar with the procedures needed to obtain blood, where a small needle is inserted into a vein and a vile of blood is drawn. Blood collection is minimally painful and, when done right, is virtually painless. While blood can be tested for multiple abnormalities, the most common investigations in IBS look for anemia and glandular problems like hypo- or hyperthyroidism. Blood electrolytes such as calcium and potassium will also be tested to see if they are abnormal, because derangements in electrolytes can cause bowel dysfunction or be caused by bowel dysfunction.

Barium Enema

Barium is a radiopaque substance that is easily visualized by X-ray. A barium enema allows a radiologist to measure the size of the bowel and see lesions that may be causing symptoms. Measuring the bowel's diameter is important to diagnose megacolon, an abnormal dilation of the bowel. While the test may not be as accurate as sigmoidoscopy or colonoscopy, for simple complaints like isolated constipation without warning signs it may be the test of choice.

SIGMOIDOSCOPY

Many doctors believe that a sigmoidoscopy is necessary for evaluating IBS. Flexible sigmoidoscopy involves the insertion of a thin, flexible tube inside the rectum and descending colon. During the exam, you will be asked to lie on your side with knees drawn into your chest. Prior to inserting the lubricated sigmoidoscope, the doctor will perform a rectal exam. Depending on your doctor's procedures and your own preferences, you may be able to watch the procedure on a video monitor. During the procedure, if your doctor finds an abnormal lesion in the bowel, expect him to take biopsies. Also, if a colonic polyp is identified, a common and usually benign finding, it will probably be removed.

Sigmoidoscopy is often normal in IBS. Intense bowel spasms preventing the scope's progress while causing pain is one finding suggestive of IBS. In fact, there are people who cannot tolerate this procedure secondary to pain. If you are experiencing significant pain during the procedure, let your doctor know. Complications are rare with sigmoidoscopy; however, bleeding, infection, and perforation can occur.

The test takes fifteen to forty-five minutes to perform and can be mildly uncomfortable. For most people, however, the worst part about flexible sigmoidoscopy is the bowel preparation the night before. In order for the doctor to assess any abnormalities, the bowel has to be totally clean. Your doctor will instruct you to fast overnight and use one or more enemas, coupled with drinking a special fluid to cleanse the bowel. Some physicians will not order an enema since this can cause distortions in the bowel that can make interpretation difficult. Nevertheless, expect to spend some time in the bathroom the evening and morning before the test. Without a doubt, for most people, this is the most uncomfortable part of the exam. My suggestion is that between bowel movements you take a hot sitz bath for five to twenty minutes to help relieve anorectal irritation. Rather than wiping, shower after a bowel movement, as showering is much less abrasive and irritating.

The advantage to a flexible sigmoidoscopy is that the test is quick, and most people don't require sedation. If you want sedation, you should inform your doctor prior to the test's being ordered, as sedation usually means the procedure has to be done in the hospital rather than in the doctor's office. However, flexible sigmoidoscopy can only visualize the most terminal part of the bowel, the descending colon, leaving two-thirds of your bowel unexamined. For this reason, many doctors prefer full colonoscopy.

Full Colonoscopy

Full colonoscopy examines the entire colon. The bowel preparation for full colonoscopy is similar to that for a flexible sigmoidoscopy. Once again, it is important to follow your physician's instructions so the bowel will be clean for the examination. With colonoscopy, sedation is often required, with the procedure usually performed in a hospital endoscopy suite. In the endoscopy suite, you will be sedated and your vital signs monitored. Like flexible sigmoidoscopy, your doctor will insert a long, flexible tube into the anus. Colonoscopy usually takes no more than one hour and, for most people, thanks to sedation, is only mildly uncomfortable.

If any abnormal tissue is seen, a biopsy will be taken and, if possible, the tissue removed. After the procedure, you will be observed until the sedation wears off, and someone will have to pick you up at the hospital since you will not be permitted to drive following the procedure.

Unlike the sigmoidoscopy, colonoscopy can visualize the entire large bowel. For this reason, many physicians consider colonoscopy superior to sigmoidoscopy. One of the reasons why I prefer full colonoscopy is that, during the procedure, any lesions identified can be biopsied, removed, or dilated, something that may not be possible during sigmoidoscopy. Furthermore, if you have a sigmoidoscopy and a lesion is found, full colonoscopy is clearly indicated to examine the entire colon for additional lesions. Hence, when considering cost, hassle, and medical impact, full colonoscopy is probably the best choice.

Abdominal X-Ray

Otherwise known as a flat plate of the abdomen, the abdominal X-ray gives your doctor a quick look at the small and large intestine. The procedure is painless and usually no fasting or special preparation is required. There is, however, a small amount of radiation exposure. Abdominal X-rays provide a rapid evaluation of the bowel's size and gas/stool content and is often used to diagnose intestinal obstruction.

Colonic Transit Time

Measuring colonic transit evaluates the time it takes for ingested material to move through the bowel. Frequently employed to evaluate severe or recalcitrant constipation, the test involves the ingestion of a small quantity of a radiopaque marker. While some radiation exposure occurs, this procedure is relatively safe, inexpensive, simple, and accurate. After ingestion of the radiopaque material, an X-ray of the abdomen is taken five days later to see how much of the marker remains. Approximately

80 percent of the material will typically be gone in five days. A more expensive and detailed test involves the ingestion of a delayed-release capsule that contains a small amount of radioactive material. Called radioscintigraphy, this test is used to evaluate the stomach, small bowel, and the colon.

Stool Sample and Culture

If your doctor suspects that an infection is causing your symptoms, he or she may ask for a stool sample. Collecting stool probably isn't on anyone's top-ten list of favorite pastimes; however, this is an excellent test for diagnosing infection or malabsorption syndromes. Your doctor will give you specific instructions on how to collect the stool, and it's important that you deliver to your doctor's office as fresh a specimen as possible. Rapid turn-around time between collection and testing offers the best results and may preclude the need for additional samples. Try not to mix urine with the stool, as this may alter the test results.

Tests of Pelvic Floor Function

Defecation relies on a delicate balance between colonic reflexes and pelvic muscles that allow for the passage of stool. Symptoms such as excessive straining, an incomplete sense of evacuation following a bowel movement, rectal pain, manual removal of feces, or the need to support the vaginal wall in order to achieve defecation all suggest pelvic muscle dysfunction.

To measure pelvic muscle function, your doctor may ask you to expel his or her finger or a weighted balloon from your rectum. This test evaluates the puborectalis muscle, an important muscle for bowel movements. In fact, a nonrelaxing puborectalis muscle can cause constipation. Your doctor may also have you perform several additional maneuvers to see how the perineum reacts. The perineum is the area between the anus and the scrotum in men or the vagina in women.

Anorectal Manometry

This is an uncommon test that is normally reserved for suspected high or low anal sphincter tone. Elevated abnormal sphincter tone or spasm is found in anismus (the abnormal contraction of pelvic muscles), whereas low tone is common in Hirschsprung's disease, a neurological disorder of the bowel characterized by abnormal nerve development.

Defecography

This test involves the expulsion of a barium load from the bowel, which is recorded radiographically. Defecography can detect anatomic and functional abnormalities in the rectum and anus. The test is occasionally used to evaluate intractable constipation.

Proctography

Proctography utilizes radiographic images of defecation to evaluate anorectal function. Sometimes the amount of "artificial stool" a patient can expel is measured to test distal bowel function. Distal bowel function is intimately related to defecation and can affect the ability to pass a stool.

EMG (Electromyogram)

Defecation requires the coordination of nerves that supply voluntary and involuntary muscles. Nervous system disorders can cause defecation problems. EMG is used to evaluate these nerves, which can be damaged by trauma, disease, or persistent, excessive straining. This procedure is typically used to evaluate fecal incontinence. Other neurological tests may involve electrical stimulation of the rectum or magnetic stimulation of the anal nerves.

Ultrasound

Ultrasound is used to evaluate abdominal organs and to visualize anatomical defects involving the bowel or anus. Ultrasound is also employed to investigate the gallbladder, which can produce abdominal pain when diseased.

PSYCHOLOGICAL EVALUATION

Given the fact that some people with IBS may have psychological issues that impact their symptoms, do not be surprised if your physician asks you to have a psychiatric evaluation. Don't be offended if you are asked to talk to a professional about your feelings. Seeing a psychiatrist or psychologist does not mean you are crazy! The best doctors insist on a complete evaluation, and this necessitates taking care of the mind as well as the body. Furthermore, like many conditions such as heart disease, asthma, and inflammatory bowel disease, what goes on in the body can have a dramatic impact on what goes on in the mind, and vice versa. The same holds true for IBS, and talking to someone about how your symptoms have affected your feelings is a win-win situation. We'll delve deeper into the psychology of IBS in Chapter 4.

CHOOSING A DOCTOR

Most people initially turn to their primary care physician to be evaluated for IBS-related symptoms, a role that is typically played by a family practice or internal medicine doctor. Primary care physicians are an excellent place to start and can collect some basic information. If, however, you suspect you have IBS or currently carry this diagnosis, I strongly suggest a visit to a board-certified gastroenterologist. This is not to imply that family practice or internal medicine physicians cannot competently diagnose and treat IBS. In fact, as a board-certified internal medicine physician, I have successfully diagnosed and treated many patients with IBS. I am making this recommendation because gastroenterologists have the most experience in evaluating and treating this disorder. A gastroenterologist has extensive expertise and experience in one area of the body—the gut. These physicians treat IBS all the time and are usually aware of the most recent developments and treatments.

GET A SECOND OPINION

Irritable bowel is a frequently misdiagnosed syndrome. In other words, there are people diagnosed with IBS who really have something else causing their symptoms, and, conversely, there are people who really have IBS but who carry a non-IBS diagnosis. While doctors are intelligent people, they do make mistakes, and it is in your best interest to verify your diagnosis by getting a second opinion. Given its nonspecific and diverse symptoms, IBS is easy to confuse with other disorders. Unfortunately, when a doctor makes a mistake, the consequences for you can be severe. This is why it always pays to get a second opinion. You may learn that your IBS is not as severe as first suspected or discover that you don't even have IBS. A healthy dose of skepticism never hurt and will keep your doctor on his toes.

YOU HAVE IBS—WHAT'S NEXT?

So, you got a second opinion and, yes, you have IBS. What's next? First, let your doctor help you get the symptoms under control. Stabilizing your IBS is important not only because you'll feel better physically and emotionally, but also so eventually you can rid yourself of IBS. Right now, however, I suggest you trust your doctor. Your physician knows what is needed to stabilize your IBS and put control back in your hands. You may prefer not to use drugs, but if your doctor believes medication is best for right now, do as your doctor says. The simple truth is that medications, when appropriately prescribed, help far more people than they hurt. Once your symptoms have calmed down and you've learned what makes your IBS tick, then you and your physician can look at ways to control your IBS, rather than having your IBS control you.

I also recommend enlisting the services of a nutritionist. Good nutrition is the backbone of a healthy life, and studies have shown that people with IBS have inadequate intakes of several important nutrients. One study found that people with IBS had less adequate diets and a significantly lower intake of folate, ascorbic acid, and vitamin A, along with an inadequate intake of many nutrients. Besides helping to discover nutritional deficiencies, a nutritionist can help you identify foods that may help or aggravate your symptoms. Diet and IBS will be discussed in detail in Chapter 5.

OVERVIEW OF IBS TREATMENT

Once a diagnosis of IBS is made, the first step in treatment is always an extensive reassuring dialogue between the patient and healthcare provider. Your doctor will want to provide as much information as he or she can regarding IBS, as the more you know, the better you will be able to control the symptoms. Reassurance is vital because many people with IBS believe there is something terribly wrong with them. While the symptoms of IBS can be uncomfortable, the good news is that the condition is not fatal, will not reduce your life span, and with proper care can be managed or cured.

The second part of treating IBS is to best manage the symptoms. Until we know for certain what causes IBS, most healthcare practitioners will be forced to concentrate their efforts on treating the symptoms rather than on the cause. However, it is worth repeating that the Brain-Gut Model has the potential to revolutionize the way we think about IBS. Supporting this theory is the observation that in people with IBS who do not have depression or anxiety, antidepressants are often effective. This is why I recommend that a trial of antidepressant therapy be used for every individual with IBS who does not respond to conservative treatment. This antidepressant can be in the form of an alternative therapy, such as St. John's wort, or a conventional agent, such as Prozac.

It is always preferable to treat the cause of a condition rather than just the symptoms, but this is not always possible with IBS. Part of the challenge in treating IBS is that the condition has multiple causes. In other words, many roads lead to the symptoms we call IBS, and what causes IBS in one person may not cause IBS in another. What is beginning to become clear is that the constellation of symptoms referred to collectively as IBS is really the end-point of multiple pathways that may or may not be operative in every individual. Given this consideration, physicians need to treat each person as an individual, examining their total health picture and identifying those mechanisms operational in that unique individual.

While symptom-based therapy is not ideal, given the fluctuating nature of the syndrome, this is a reasonable initial approach for IBS. For instance, while most people with IBS have either diarrhea- or constipation-predominant IBS, alternating diarrhea and constipation can often be found in the same individual. As the symptoms change, it is reasonable to expect that the treatment will also change. Treating IBS often involves a delicate interplay between balancing the treatment of one symptom while trying not to create another symptom.

Clearly, the treatment of IBS is complex and challenging, with patience being required on the part of both the healthcare provider and the patient. Don't be surprised or discouraged if what worked for your symptoms one day does not work the next. At its best, the management of IBS is a dynamic process, constantly subject to revision as the syndrome changes. The bottom line is that the treatment of IBS must be individualized to achieve the best results. Because of this, a certain amount of trial and error is involved, and both you and your healthcare professional will have to be patient and learn to give each treatment an opportunity to work. While some treatments will produce measurable relief in hours to days, lasting relief is often measured in weeks to months.

And as you'll learn in this book, there are many things that you can do—change your diet and take supplements, address underlying psychological factors, start exercising, and employ alternative therapies—so that your IBS can be managed and controlled, allowing you to live the life you so richly deserve.

Chapter 4

The Psychology of IBS

For decades, many experts and patients mistakenly believed that irritable bowel syndrome was solely a psychiatric disorder. Modern research has fortunately shattered that myth, and we now know that IBS is truly characterized by dysfunctional bowel motility and sensation. While there are clearly organic mechanisms operating in IBS, there are, in fact, psychological mechanisms also at work in some people. For people who seek medical treatment for IBS, experts estimate that 50 to 90 percent have a psychiatric disorder. Psychological factors have a profound impact with respect to treatment success as well: People with anxiety and depression generally experience less improvement in abdominal pain, distention, and diarrhea.

While we cannot blame IBS entirely on emotions, it is equally clear that there are both physical and psychological processes at work. Before we examine the psychology of IBS, we have to answer one very important question: "Why should the mind play such an important role in IBS?" Thanks to recent research findings, we are now closer than ever to answering this question.

THE BRAIN-GUT MODEL

Researchers have observed that many people with IBS have autonomic nervous system dysfunction similar to that found in individuals with anxiety and depression. They have also discovered that people with IBS "share certain abnormalities in regional brain activity with posttraumatic stress disorder and depressed patients." This line of thinking has yielded some unexpected results and cutting-edge research demonstrating that the neural mechanisms characteristic of psychiatric disorders also are operational in IBS. We have also found that these dysfunctional systems stimulate each other, creating a vicious cycle of IBS, anxiety, and depression. And, surprisingly, these derangements exist and respond to treatment even in people with IBS who do not have anxiety or depression.

Our nervous system can be divided into the central nervous system (CNS) and enteric nervous system (ENS). The CNS consists of the brain and spinal cord and is in charge of virtually all our bodily functions. The ENS refers to the nerves within the bowel. While the CNS retains significant control over the ENS, the ENS also clearly influences the CNS.

The ENS and CNS, from a developmental perspective, are derived from the same embryonic material group of cells. Given this consideration, it is not surprising that they influence each other. Both the CNS and ENS have "adaptive neuronal plasticity," or the capacity to learn new information, and these systems also share neurotransmitters, chemicals responsible for transmitting nerve signals between nerve endings and bodily organs.

Researchers have discovered that several CNS nuclei that control the bowel "also coordinate emotional, physiologic, and fear-conditioning reactions to perceived danger as components of the innate 'fear circuit.'" The CNS controls the "fear circuit" through stress chemicals like adrenaline and corticotropin-releasing factor. Perhaps the most dramatic example of this fear circuit is the "fight-or-flight," or stress response, which has a dramatic impact on the bowel, shutting down the stomach and increasing colonic activity. Experts believe that fear circuit dysfunction is involved in conditions like posttraumatic stress disorder and anxiety. Many different CNS regions are involved in the fear circuit and routinely receive information from the ENS.

Brain-Gut Model

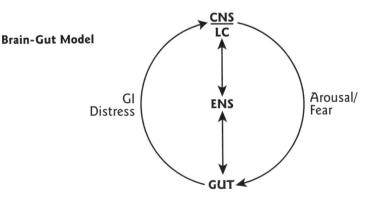

Used by permission: Elsevier. From Lydiard BR, Falsetti SA. Experience with anxiety and depression treatment studies: implications for designing irritable bowel syndrome clinical trials. *Am J Med* 1999;107 (Suppl 5): 65–73.

One of the more important nuclei in this fear circuit is called the locus ceruleus (LC). Experimental studies have demonstrated that the LC is stimulated by colonic distention, and this causes the LC to send excitatory signals to the rest of the CNS. It is theorized that people with IBS have a dysfunctional fear circuit that connects the CNS and ENS and results in the symptoms we call IBS. Specifically, input from the ENS travels to the LC and results in increased CNS arousal that in turn causes gastrointestinal (GI) symptoms. Normally, this fear circuit is either dampened or turned off, only being used when truly needed. In IBS, a cycle of persistent CNS and ENS stimulation may occur, each system feeding off the other, resulting in continuous arousal.

Now, how does this Brain-Gut Model tie into IBS being both a physical and psychological condition? Research has shown that psychiatric medications can help people with IBS, regardless of whether or not they have a psychiatric disorder. In fact, we suspect that these agents "normalize" the brain's fear circuit. This same mechanism is also theorized to play a role in the success of "cognitive-behavioral" therapy, which reduces hyperreactivity to visceral and emotional stimuli in IBS. This means that psychological interventions, both conventional and alternative, may provide a great deal of relief for those with IBS.

STRESS CHEMICALS AND IBS

Intimately related to the fear circuit are chemicals that mediate stress reactions. These stress reactions can be either physical or emotional, and involve a system called the "hypothalamic-pituitary-adrenal axis." When we are presented with a stressful situation, it is first recognized by the hypothalamus, a structure deep within the brain. The hypothalamus sends a signal to the pituitary gland, which sends a signal to the adrenal glands. The adrenal glands sit on top of the kidneys and secrete hormones, known as glucocorticoids, that help the body adapt to stress. A major chemical mediator of the ENS-CNS fear circuit is corticotropin-releasing factor (CRF). In the presence of stress, the hypothalamus releases CRF, which triggers the hypothalamic-pituitary-adrenal axis. Equally important, CRF is involved in pain perception, produces anxiety, and can influence the LC.

Researchers speculate that derangements in how the CNS, ENS, and CRF interact play a vital role in IBS. Each of these systems regulates bowel function and how the CNS interprets bowel function. These complex inter-relations, coupled with the fact that CRF can produce anxiety, may be the reason why people with depression or anxiety often have nonspecific bowel complaints that are similar to those seen in IBS. The fact that IBS is more common in women may also be explained by interactions between CRF and the hypothalamic-pituitary-adrenal axis system. Research has shown that, in women, the hypothalamic-pituitary-adrenal axis exhibits a more intense and persistent reaction than seen in men. We also know that estrogen causes an increase in cortisol secretion, accompanied by a greater response to stress.

How does this relate to irritable bowel? In people without IBS, these stress-bowel pathways shut down once a crisis is over. In people with IBS, for reasons that remain unclear, these stress-bowel pathways do not shut down and ultimately lock into a self-perpetuating cycle of bowel hypersensitivity—increased pain, anxiety, and depression, which leads to further bowel complaints.

The fear circuit can influence IBS and dramatically affect the symptoms on both a conscious and unconscious level. Researchers suspect that in some people with IBS, this self-perpetuating fear circuit may stem from a traumatic event. IBS symptoms are then continually triggered by "numerous environmental cues, which may remind them consciously or unconsciously of that trauma, [and] might exacerbate their symptoms via conditioned fear pathways that modify intestinal functioning."

An example will make this clear. We know that people with IBS have a high incidence of sexual abuse during childhood. It is theorized that the acute physical and emotional trauma associated with sexual abuse entrain the CNS and ENS to establish a hyperactive fear circuit in response. The sexual abuse, especially when repetitive, makes bowel pain receptors hypersensitive, and a response becomes "hardwired" into the ENS and CNS and never completely shuts off.

Later, when this individual experiences a stressful situation, the bowel "remembers" and associates this stress with previous sexual trauma, producing symptoms of IBS. However, since the pathways that control the bowels are also related to psychological disturbances, these pathways also trigger anxiety and depression. In other words, the symptoms we call IBS are actually a learned response to stress, involving a vicious cycle of bowel hypersensitivity, anxiety, and depression.

Clearly, sexual abuse is an extreme example of this mechanism. It is suspected, however, that in some people with IBS, their bowels become trained to behave a certain way when subjected to emotional stress. The intensity of this response may have its roots in the initial events that first entrained the bowel. The more traumatic the initial precipitating event, the more severe the IBS. Once again, this may not be operative in all people with IBS; however, we know that people with IBS who have a history of sexual abuse tend to have more severe symptoms that are difficult to treat.

This may also explain why many people with IBS never seek medical attention and why psychiatric symptoms are more common in those who do. In people who never seek medical attention, the precipitating events that entrained their bowel may not have been sufficient to produce severe symptoms. In those who seek medical care, the events were of sufficient intensity to permanently and severely perturb these systems and establish the vicious cycle of bowel complaints we call IBS.

Not every person with a history of sexual abuse has IBS, nor does every person with IBS have a history of sexual abuse or a psychiatric disorder. In some individuals, genetics could make their CNS-ENS systems more resistant to stress-induced derangements, but this is largely speculative. However, we do know that genetics play a large role in our resistance or susceptibility to disease. While there remains much to be learned about brain-gut interactions and IBS, there nevertheless appears to be a self-perpetuating cycle of anxiety and depression increasing the severity of IBS symptoms, while IBS increases anxiety and especially depression.

These brain-gut interactions, while being actively investigated, are supported by multiple findings. We know, for instance, that bowels become increasingly sensitive to unpleasant stimuli and that this increased sensitivity can persist for extended periods of time. According to one study, ENS neurons can be permanently sensitized by stress or other noxious stimulation. We also know that CRF probably has a role in chronic pain syndromes. These findings may in part explain why people with IBS are more sensitive to bowel stimuli. There is also active research into pharmacological agents that block CRF receptors, which may one day represent powerful new weapons in treating IBS.

With respect to victims of sexual abuse, this theory may explain why these individuals have unexplained chronic pelvic pain and painful sexual intercourse, a common finding also seen in IBS. Once again, while such generalizations do not apply to everyone with IBS, there is an accumulating body of evidence that CNS and ENS derangements—neurobiological factors involving brain-gut interactions, anxiety, and depression—may be responsible for the psychiatric complications seen in IBS.

PSYCHOLOGICAL FACTORS IN IBS

While there is much to learn regarding mind-bowel interactions, the Brain-Gut Model helps explain some of the psychological findings seen in IBS. Irritable bowel is, however, not unique, and most medical conditions result from a complex interplay between mind and body. Many illnesses can be made worse or better by how a person feels emotionally. For example, the association between asthma severity and emotions has been extensively documented. The same can be said about heart disease—for some people, strong emotions can prove deadly.

The bowel, being normally sensitive to stress, is hypersensitive in people with IBS. In fact, we have known since the 1950s that emotions impact the bowel, when it was found that people who were hostile or angry had increased spastic bowel activity. Conversely, people who are depressed can have decreased bowel contractions. Similar findings have been reported in people with IBS.

While this mind-body connection is active in many diseases, IBS has the unfortunate history of being labeled as a purely "psychological" illness. Multiple theories add to the confusion surrounding the exact role that psychology plays in IBS, variously blaming personality defects, dependent relationships with parents, anger, or an overemphasis on potty training and bowel habits in childhood.

Nevertheless, we do know that some people who suffer from IBS also have to contend with psychological disorders. Studies show a high prevalence of psychological symptoms in IBS patients and suggest that psychological factors play an important role in the pathogenesis of the illness in many people.

As discussed earlier, there is a well-established correlation between IBS and a history of sexual or physical abuse. One study found that 55 percent of patients with IBS reported a history of sexual abuse, compared to only 5 percent of those with inflammatory bowel disease. In addition, a history of abuse can directly impact the severity of IBS-related symptoms, including symptomatic pain, functional impairment, and poor treatment results. Functional gastrointestinal disorders like IBS are also more common in people with a history of posttraumatic stress disorder, and, as mentioned previously, several authors have concluded that trauma might play a role in the etiology of IBS.

Many experts also believe that, for some people, irritable bowel syndrome is a disorder in which anxiety is focused on an "internal stimulus," namely the gut. Early in the course of IBS, it is suspected that anxiety predominates, whereas in chronic IBS depression is more common. We also know that people with anxiety or panic disorders tend to have an increased risk of IBS. Panic disorder is a form of anxiety in which the individual experiences a sudden and unprovoked sensation of extreme anxiety and fear, with feelings of impending doom, which is often coupled with increased respiration and heart rate. Several studies have found that panic disorder may be associated with IBS and that people with mood disorders like depression have an increased risk of IBS.

While these findings are accurate for some individuals with IBS, they do not tell the whole story. As with most illnesses, what goes on in the body often affects the mind, and vice versa—IBS is no exception. IBS involves both physical and psychological manifestations, and individuals with IBS often score higher on psychological tests that measure for psychiatric disorders. Multiple studies document a strong relationship between bowel disorders and psychological/social problems.

In some people with IBS, psychiatric problems precede or begin at about the same time as IBS. One study found that in 77 percent of those surveyed, a major psychiatric disorder came before or coincided with the initial IBS symptoms. These researchers also found that people with IBS had a higher incidence of depression and anxiety. It has also been observed that some people with IBS think more about illness and experience a higher rate of disability. In fact, one study found that those with IBS had more concerns about their health when compared to people with depression. Common worries included concerns about having cancer or that their symptoms represented a potentially serious illness. These concerns can have a dramatic impact on IBS and often contribute to poor treatment response. Other factors that lead to poor treatment outcomes include lack of psychosocial support, a finding not uncommon to multiple medical disorders, as social functioning impacts the severity and course of the condition.

Some authorities believe that IBS may, for some people, be a learned response that has been reinforced through secondary gain. Illness and "sick behavior" are in part learned behaviors, with different cultures displaying their own attitudes regarding illness. In many societies, being ill confers a social advantage, such as increased attention from significant others and temporary relief from work duties. We do know that some people, either intentionally or unintentionally, exploit sick-role behavior for these gains. This sick-role behavior can range from a child who "plays" sick so he or she can have a day off from school to Munchausen syndrome, a disorder in which people present complaints and undergo invasive tests and surgery in order to achieve secondary gain. Many authorities suspect that, in some people with IBS, seeking secondary gain through illness is operating at an unconscious level.

Studies have shown that the way a child learns to report and display illness can impact his or her health as an adult. We learn how to assume an appropriate sick role from our culture and our parents. It has been shown that "reinforcement and modeling of gastrointestinal illness behavior during childhood are significantly correlated with having a diagnosis of IBS as an adult." For some individuals, IBS may be part of a response learned in childhood.

But do psychological symptoms cause IBS or does IBS cause psychological symptoms?—a gastroenterological chicken-or-the-egg kind of question. While we know that anxiety and depression are more common in IBS, we also know that anxiety and depression can make IBS worse. Adding to the confusion is that even in normal people bowel function is sensitive to emotional stimuli. While many studies examine these questions, their results are often contradictory. What has emerged, however, is that the relationship between IBS and the mind is a two-way street: For many people, emotions influence how their bowels react, and their bowels influence how their minds react.

What is important to remember is that there is no simple explanation for IBS. While it is certainly not fair to say that IBS is a purely psychological disorder, a physician would be remiss not to consider psychological factors when evaluating IBS. While psychological factors may not play a role in every case of IBS, when they are present, psychiatric symptoms impact the course of the syndrome.

One of the most important lessons you can learn from this book is that the more you know about IBS, the more you will be able to successfully manage the syndrome. Many people with IBS become defensive when confronted with the possibility that their symptoms may in part be related to how they feel emotionally. I strongly believe, however, that it's important to keep an open mind and explore all the possibilities. What I hope this book will teach you is to ask the right questions. Questions about your symptoms: What makes them worse? What makes them better? Questions about your diet, and the foods or medications you take. I also want you to ask questions about how you feel inside. The more we understand how we feel, the better we can cope with those issues that make us feel the way we do. According to one group of experts, "Those patients who accept that stress may contribute to their IBS symptoms tend to have a more favorable outcome than those who attribute symptoms solely to physical illness. It is helpful for patients to understand why they have their symptoms and what makes them worse."

STRESS AND IBS

Multiple studies have documented that stress can exacerbate IBS. A major limitation of this research is that stress-induced alterations in gut motility are found even in people who do not have IBS. Studies have also shown that bowel distention can cause "distress" that is made worse under experimental stress conditions. The question is, which stress-induced alterations in bowel motility are abnormal, and which are normal?

As indicated previously, we know that IBS often appears after a stressful event, and studies have found that the onset of IBS is occasionally associated with extremely traumatic, "life-threatening" events. Equally compelling, research has also shown that experiencing a life-threatening event can result in months of gastrointestinal symptoms.

Overall, researchers have found that people with IBS report an increased number of stressful events when compared with the rest of the population. One of the problems with these studies, however, is that most of these trials are retrospective and influenced by how accurately people remember stressful events. Equally problematic is the fact that when ill, people want to identify a precipitating event. Human beings, by their very nature, seek causality. It is more psychologically comforting to blame our ills on a specific precipitant rather than accept the fact that good and bad life events often occur by random chance.

Plus, given the fact that stress is a daily part of life, how do we evaluate the true impact of stress on IBS? I suspect that most of us can describe at least five stressful events that occurred over the past three days. Given how common stress is, scientists are hard-pressed to definitively conclude that such a ubiquitous life event is responsible for IBS. For instance, many of you can probably recall a stressful event that exacerbated your IBS but also remember a time when you were stressed but remained symptom free. How do we know that an IBS exacerbation would or would not have occurred regardless of the presence of stress?

Now, it is not my intention to conclude that stress has nothing to do with IBS. Clearly, there are many excellent studies that demonstrate with reasonable scientific certainly that stress can exacerbate IBS. The point is that, when critically examined, the relationship between stress and IBS is not a simple one. To highlight these difficulties, it is worthwhile to examine one study that exemplifies the complexity of stress and IBS.

This prospective study, from the Department of Psychology at the University of East London, examined thirty individuals with IBS over five weeks to see if "hassles" and "uplifts" (positive events) had any impact on their symptoms. These researchers found that both positive and negative emotions had little impact on the severity of IBS symptoms, but total symptoms were found to be "significantly associated with hassles in the following weeks." In other words, IBS severity determined how people felt emotionally—those who had significant IBS symptoms were destined to feel worse emotionally the following week. The study concluded that there was a cumulative effect of symptoms: An increase in symptom severity was associated with an increase in stress, but more hassles alone did not appear to exacerbate symptoms. Conversely, the researchers also concluded that there was no association at all between positive events and IBS symptoms. In the final analysis, the authors speculated that "IBS may not be a homogenous disorder; there may be several causes of symptoms [and] stress may be a causal or trigger factor for some sufferers. For others, symptoms may be due to other reasons." This is an important finding that is being increasingly echoed by an emerging body of literature and healthcare practitioners as well.

TREATING IBS WITH PSYCHOTHERAPY

For many individuals, psychotherapy is an effective treatment that reduces emotional pain and helps relieve irritable bowel symptoms. Most physicians will recommend psychotherapy to individuals who have a clear psychiatric condition or who do not respond to first-line medical therapy. My recommendation, however, is that an individual with any chronic condition—asthma, diabetes, heart failure, or IBS—should speak to a therapist regarding his or her feelings. Given the strong association between IBS and emotions, I emphatically recommend that everyone with IBS consult a trained professional about their feelings. Not only will talking help you feel better, there is also a strong consensus in the medical community that recognition and treatment of anxiety and depression may prevent the progression of both mental and gastrointestinal symptoms. IBS patients may benefit from acknowledging the involvement of stress and other psychological factors in perpetuating the syndrome.

I want to reiterate, however, that this does not imply that your symptoms are "all in your head." Rather, my recommendation is based on the knowledge that people who talk about their medical conditions often do better regardless of whether or not their condition is purely physical, psychological, or a combination of both. For instance, studies have demonstrated that treating both physical and emotional symptoms in IBS helps more than 50 percent of participants.

One study compared twelve weeks of conversational exploratory psychotherapy with medical treatment versus supportive listening with medical treatment in a group of 102 men and women with chronic IBS. In the women, psychotherapy was found to be superior to supportive listening in improving both physical and psychological symptoms. In the men, though a similar trend was observed, it did not achieve statistical significance. Those individuals who continued to participate in psychotherapy once the trial concluded experienced a marked improvement in their symptoms. The endpoints measured included abdominal symptoms and pain, the impact these symptoms had on daily life, the rating of a gastroenterologist, and several psychological measures. All of these improved significantly in the treatment group by the end of the trial.

The authors noted that the number of patients in the treatment group who warranted a psychiatric diagnosis fell dramatically following treatment, from thirty to only five at three months, whereas sixteen of the control group still had psychiatric illness afterward. At a follow-up one year later, the patients who had received psychotherapy remained well, but patients who had dropped out of the study had severe symptoms, and most of those in the control group who had declined psychotherapy had relapsed. Thus, patients who had dealt with the psychological issues of their IBS were able to maintain their improvements in health after treatment. In other words, improvement in psychological status led to a dramatic improvement in bowel symptoms, particularly in those who had symptoms unresponsive to standard medical treatment.

A British randomized, controlled clinical trial examined 102 people with IBS who had failed standard medical therapy. These individuals represented some of the most challenging IBS cases, with 30 percent suffering from major depression and another 18 percent having anxiety disorder.

From a physician's perspective, these are the most difficult people to treat and represent a population that is often recalcitrant to standard medical treatment. They were divided into two groups: One received standard medical therapy and the other received standard medical therapy with psychotherapy (focusing on life events related to IBS onset, such as marital discord) and relaxation training.

After three months, there was a "significantly greater improvement" in the psychotherapy group in severity of diarrhea and abdominal pain. With respect to subjective complaints, improvement of abdominal bloating was also recorded, but these results did not reach statistical significance. The people who benefited most from psychotherapy were those who had "overt psychiatric symptoms" and intermittent pain made worse by stress, particularly those individuals who came to recognize that stress exacerbated their symptoms. Not only did the treatment group benefit physically, they also experienced significant improvement in anxiety and depression. Again, improvement in psychological status lessened IBS symptoms. Also, in a one-year follow-up, the group who had undergone psychotherapy maintained their improvements.

While we cannot say that psychological factors are always involved, studies like these demonstrate that anxiety and depression are a factor in bowel dysfunction in some patients with IBS. Most illnesses are characterized by a complex interplay between mind and body. For instance, no one can say that cancer is caused by "bad thoughts." But few people would deny that having cancer profoundly impacts how one feels emotionally, and one's emotions can greatly affect the outcome of the disease. The same is true for people with heart disease, asthma, and IBS—the body impacts the mind and the mind impacts the body.

Talking to a professional is not an admission of mental illness; rather, it is a way to help you better deal with your symptoms and determine if how you think is affecting the way your bowels feel. After examining the literature, there is little doubt that psychotherapy is a powerful adjunct in treating IBS. For many with irritable bowel, even if there is not a psychiatric disorder present, the mind-body connection can best be managed with the aid of a trained professional. Equally important in dealing with psychological issues is to involve family members in the therapeutic process. You are not alone in your suffering, and what affects you also affects your family. Open communication between you, your family, and a caring therapist is clearly one of several first steps you will need to take on your road to recovery. While the length of psychotherapy required varies from individual to individual, there is ample evidence that psychotherapy can help people with IBS. Talking to people will not only help your symptoms, but can also help reduce the sense of helplessness some people feel when confronted by IBS.

SUPPORT GROUPS AND OTHER RESOURCES

There is little doubt that being diagnosed with irritable bowel syndrome is disturbing for most individuals. Fortunately, many communities sponsor support groups where people with IBS can develop friendships with others who understand their experiences and frustrations. Some people with chronic medical conditions make the mistake of withdrawing from the world. This is a potentially tragic error, since humans by their very nature are social, and engaging in positive interactions with others is necessary for survival. Studies show that positive social contacts also protect against disease and death. And as we learned earlier, people with IBS who are lonely or socially isolated often have poor outcomes and tend to experience the most severe disease. Evidence indicates that support groups can greatly help people with gastrointestinal disorders.

If you want to learn more about IBS support groups in your area, call the Digestive Disease Clearinghouse, which is also one of the best sources for general information and breaking news on IBS:

Digestive Disease Clearinghouse
2 Information Way
Bethesda, MD 20892-3570
Phone: 800-891-5389 or 301-654-3810
Fax: 301-907-8906
Website: www.health.gov/nhic/NHICScripts/Entry.cfm? HRCode=HR0986

Organized in 1987, the Irritable Bowel Syndrome Association is dedicated to helping IBS sufferers find patient support groups, treatment information, and other educational materials:

IBS Association
1440 Whalley Avenue #145
New Haven, CT 06515
Website: www.ibsassociation.org

The International Foundation for Functional Gastrointestinal Disorders (IFFGD) is a nonprofit education organization providing information, assistance, and support to people affected by gastrointestinal disorders:

IFFGD
P.O. Box 170864
Milwaukee, WI 53217-8076
Phone: 414-964-1799
Fax: 414-964-7176
Website: www.aboutibs.org

If you're looking for an excuse to surf the Web, there are several excellent on-line IBS resources, a few of which are listed below.

- An excellent website where you can find information on IBS support groups is www.digitalabstract.net/irritablebowelsyndrome/ibssupport-groups.asp.

- An extensive database for IBS, with original articles, chat rooms, and links to information about medications, diet, and symptoms, can be found at www.ibscrohns.about.com.

- HealingWell.com has an IBS resource center that offers chat rooms as well as information, community message boards, newsletters, books, and a host of IBS related links: members.aol.com/ibswebpage/ibs.htm.

- The IBS Voice has useful links, including an IBS self-help group: www.drugvoice.com/ibs.htm.

- The National Institute of Diabetes and Digestive and Kidney Diseases (part of the National Institutes of Health) has an extensive website loaded with useful information: www. niddk.nih.gov/health/digest/pubs/irrbowel/irrbowel.htm.

Sexual and physical abuse can be devastating, and here is a small sampling of the available resources:

The Rape, Abuse, and Incest National Network (RAINN) is a leading anti–sexual assault organization that offers information, counseling center locations, and a 24-hour hotline that is free and confidential:

Rape, Abuse & Incest National Network
635-B Pennsylvania Avenue, SE

Washington, DC 20003
Sexual Assault Hotline: 800-656-HOPE (4673)
Phone: 202-544-1034
Fax: 202-544-3556
Website: www.rainn.org

Woman in Need is a group devoted to the empowerment of women who are victims of physical or sexual abuse. WIN has an established referral network to direct women to the appropriate local agencies for assistance:

Women in Need, Inc.
3431 Garden City Boulevard, SE
Roanoke, VA 24014
Phone: 540-427-5250
Fax: 540-427-2515
Website: www.win-foundation.org/index.shtml

The Sexual Abuse Support Home Page offers helpful information:

Sexual Abuse Support Home Page
Website: sasupport.healthyplace2.com.

Chapter 5

Diet and Irritable Bowel

S ome people with irritable bowel will have to change the way they eat and live. The good news is that these changes will help you not only to better control your symptoms, but also to live a longer and healthier life. The bad news is that you may have to give up some the foods you love. In this chapter, we'll look at how food allergies or sensitivities contribute to IBS. In addition, we'll find out what foods or food additives to avoid if you have IBS and what foods you should increase.

FOOD ALLERGIES AND INTOLERANCES

It is estimated that about 2 percent of adults have food allergies, and many authorities believe that food allergies and intolerances are to blame for some cases of IBS. Food allergies can cause depression in susceptible individuals, which is also of interest to people with IBS. First, let's define our terms. A *food allergy or hypersensitivity* is a reaction to a specific food that is the result of an immune, allergy-related mechanism. Conversely, a *food intolerance or sensitivity* is defined as a nonallergic, "unpleasant reaction" to food.

While the exact association between food and IBS remains elusive, many people with IBS avoid certain foods because they believe a particular food makes their symptoms worse. While anyone with IBS can have a food allergy or intolerance, one study found that people with diarrhea-predominant IBS had the most adverse reactions to food. Moreover, people with diarrhea-predominant IBS respond better to food elimination diets, and a significant number of them experience symptom relief while on an elimination diet.

For a variety of reasons, the impact of adverse food reactions is diffi-

Common Allergenic Foods

- Alcohol
- Milk
- Eggs
- Caffeine
- Wheat
- Sorbitol
- Fatty foods
- Corn
- Sulfites
- Gas-producing vegetables (particularly broccoli, Brussels sprouts, cabbage, cauliflower, onions)

cult to assess in IBS. Part of the difficulty is determining the true incidence of food reactions. Studies estimate that the prevalence of food intolerance in gastrointestinal disorders is 16 to 33 percent; however, many experts concede that food allergies are probably significantly underdiagnosed.

Perhaps the only general recommendation regarding food allergies and IBS is to avoid foods you know will cause an exacerbation of your symptoms. While almost any food can be blamed, the most common offenders are alcohol, caffeine, fatty foods, milk, wheat, corn, eggs, gas-producing vegetables (particularly broccoli, Brussels sprouts, cabbage, cauliflower, and onions), and sorbitol (an artificial sweetener found in sugarless food). As an aside, since alcohol and tobacco can act as gastrointestinal irritants, people with IBS should avoid alcohol and tobacco products.

Food allergies can be caused by the food itself or by something artificial in the food, such as a coloring or preserving agent. Unfortunately, food colorings or dyes are used almost everywhere, so it's important to read food (and drug) labels to see if a food coloring is present. Sulfites are used as preservatives and are quite common in both medicines and foods. Common sulfiting agents include potassium bisulfite, potassium metabisulfite, sodium bisulfite, sodium sulfite, and sulfur dioxide. Sulfites can hide anywhere from the salad bar to your favorite wine.

In a food allergy, when a person consumes an offending food, multiple allergic mediators are released into the bowel, which cause symptoms similar to IBS. Food allergies or hypersensitivities are mediated by immunoglobulin E (IgE), the chief antibody of the allergic response that we also see operating in seasonal allergies. It is the job of IgE to recognize and form an antibody-antigen interaction with allergens like pollen and dander. Sometimes, however, IgE becomes sensitive to specific proteins in food, thereby triggering an allergic reaction that involves immune cells, such as mast cells and basophils. These cells release chemicals (histamine and prostaglandins) into the bowel that result in smooth muscle contraction and increased fluid secretion. As we know, it is suspected that abnormal smooth muscle contraction is responsible for IBS-related abdominal pain. Likewise, increased intestinal fluid is a basic mechanism behind diarrhea. This allergic reaction to food causes a symptom complex remarkably similar to the one in IBS.

Food intolerances are not immune mediated and commonly result from an enzymatic deficiency. The prototypical food intolerance is lactose intolerance, where there is a deficiency in the enzyme that digests lactose. Hence, when lactose enters the bowel, it acts like an osmotic laxative, drawing fluid into the bowel and potentially causing diarrhea/cramps, symptoms common to IBS.

One study found that specific foods provoked symptoms in fourteen of twenty-one patients who carried a diagnosis of IBS. Food intolerance was subsequently identified in six of these patients. The researchers found significantly elevated rectal levels of prostaglandin-2 (PGE2), which plays a role in the body's inflammatory response and in diseases such as inflammatory bowel disease (IBD) and asthma. It is suspected that in IBD, prostaglandins are responsible for the diarrhea. One group of authors concluded that food intolerance appeared to be very important in the pathogenesis of IBS. Some of the foods identified by this study were wheat, corn, dairy products, coffee, tea, and citrus fruits. Now, don't go eliminating these foods from your diet! Food allergies and intolerances are highly individualized, and what may cause symptoms in one person may not cause any symptoms in you.

Another study examined twenty-seven patients with IBS using exclusion diets and a double-blind food challenge. Only three subjects were found to have a food hypersensitivity that was responsible for their symptoms. But these individuals were also reported to have positive skin tests to common inhalant allergens and atopy, both markers of allergic sensitization. While this study does not offer strong support to the theory that food hypersensitivities are a major cause of IBS, it does indicate that in certain individuals, food allergies can play a role, especially in those who are predisposed to allergic illness. The possibility of food hypersensitivity should probably always be considered in the treatment of IBS, particularly in the presence of other allergy-related manifestations.

These studies demonstrate the complex interplay between allergies and IBS, and it is sometimes difficult to determine exactly which disorder is causing the symptoms. These findings also imply that food intolerances may play a larger role in IBS than actual immune-mediated food allergies. Given how common allergies and intolerances are, it is certainly reasonable to conclude that in a subgroup of people with IBS, food allergies and intolerances play a role. However, the literature in not conclusive on how large a role food allergies or intolerances play in IBS. Further complicating the picture is that alterations in gut motility can occur even by telling a patient that they have been given a food to which they think they are sensitive. Indeed, there are individuals who cannot tolerate certain foods for psychological reasons. Another complicating feature of food intolerance is that these reactions may be delayed, which makes it difficult to trace the reaction back to the food that caused it.

Despite these complications, there is adequate evidence to assert that food allergies and intolerances are operating in certain individuals with IBS. Many patients report an exacerbation of symptoms after food ingestion. Whether or not adverse reactions to foods are the key factor in making IBS symptoms worse remains to be proven. Given the fact that IBS is a heterogeneous syndrome with multiple underlying causes, it is reasonable to conclude that for some people with IBS, especially those with diarrhea-predominant IBS, food allergies and intolerances play a role and should be investigated and treated.

DIAGNOSIS AND TREATMENT OF FOOD ALLERGIES

The diagnosis of a food allergy or hypersensitivity relies on the medical history and food-allergy testing, either by the skin prick test or a blood RAST (radio-allergosorbent test). In RAST testing, a blood sample is checked for a specific IgE level. Allergies are usually indicated if an elevated IgE level is identified for a specific allergen, such as a food. If you suspect that food may be causing your symptoms, it is also critical that you keep a food diary. This information can be included in your standard IBS diary and would normally include a careful recording of what you eat and any symptoms you experience. For example, if every time you have a milkshake your IBS flares, then perhaps it would be best to forsake milkshakes. Expect your physician, dietician, or nutritionist to ask you to keep a food diary. As a rule, the more data, the better, so it's important to list everything you eat as well as your symptoms. After a period of six to eight weeks, meet with your healthcare provider, who will review the diary with you. As you can imagine, two months of recording every meal and snack demands dedication; however, the effort is rewarded if an offending food is identified.

If a specific food is found to be suspect, you will be asked to not eat that food—this is known as a food elimination diet. At a later date, you will be given that food to see if it once again causes symptoms. Known as food challenge, this is an important test not only to see if that particular food exacerbates your IBS, but also to make sure you don't unnecessarily eliminate foods you could otherwise enjoy. Food challenges can be either open, closed, or double-blinded, which means you may or may not know what food you are eating. The best challenges employ a double-blind placebo-controlled approach where neither the tester nor the subject know which is the test food and which is placebo. Just in case you're wondering how someone cannot tell what they're eating, the food or placebo is disguised in a capsule. While not perfect, elimination diets can help identify food reactions. One meta-analysis on food elimination diets in people with IBS found that they identified an offending food up to 57 percent of the time.

SORBITOL AND FRUCTOSE

Sugar malabsorption is common among people with and without IBS and can cause symptoms in both groups. Sugars like sorbitol, fructose, lactose, and sucrose are not rapidly absorbed by the bowel and create an osmotic effect by drawing water into the bowel that can, in turn, cause diarrhea. Sweeteners like fructose and sorbitol can also increase intestinal gas. Fructose and sorbitol are found naturally in fruits, and sorbitol is a common ingredient in "sugar-free" or diabetic foods and some medications. With the exception of sucrose, these sugars are often not completely absorbed even in people with perfectly normal gastrointestinal tracts.

Several studies have found that sorbitol and fructose can exacerbate IBS (although even people without IBS can react to these sweeteners as well). One study examined sugar intolerance in twenty-five individuals with IBS and twelve healthy control subjects. Several sugars were tested, including lactose, fructose, sorbitol, and sucrose, alone and in combination. The authors found that sugar malabsorption was high in both patients and control subjects, with malabsorption of at least one sugar in more than 90 percent of subjects and multiple sugar intolerances reported in several people. Not unexpectedly, people with IBS had more severe symptoms when compared with healthy subjects. Individuals who were diagnosed with a sugar intolerance were placed on an elimination diet, and 30 percent showed a "substantial improvement" in symptoms. The study concluded that "sugar malabsorption may be implicated in the development of abdominal distress in at least a subset of patients with functional bowel disorder."

A study of people without IBS found that following ingestion of 10 grams of sorbitol, an amount of sugar equal to that found in two medium pears, 10 percent had "moderate discomfort" and 17 percent had "severe discomfort." The symptoms were similar to those seen in people with IBS, with complaints of abdominal pain, diarrhea, and bloating that lasted for up to six hours following sorbitol ingestion.

These findings indicate that reactions to sugars may play a role in some people with IBS. So, you may want to eliminate sugar and artificial sweeteners from your diet for a month to see how your bowels react. These sugars are ubiquitous in processed foods but are normally listed on food labels, making them relatively easy to avoid.

LACTOSE INTOLERANCE

People who are lactose intolerant do not have enough lactase, the enzyme needed to digest lactose, a sugar found in milk. Consequently, lactose remains in the bowel and creates an osmotic effect and produces diarrhea. People with lactase deficiency complain of having diarrhea after consuming dairy products, most commonly milk and ice cream; however, people with severe lactose intolerance may not even be able to eat cheese. The condition ranges from mild to severe and tends to be more common as a person ages. As adults, about 50 percent of Hispanics, 20 percent of Caucasians, and most African-Americans have lactose intolerance. There is also an association between lactose intolerance and depression in women.

The symptoms of lactose intolerance are similar to those of irritable bowel syndrome and include diarrhea, gas, and abdominal pain. Lactose-intolerant people can also be intolerant of other common sugars, particularly sucrose, lactulose, and fructose. Particularly relevant to IBS, studies have found that lactose intolerance is significantly more common in people with IBS than in the general population, and people with IBS also appear to be more sensitive to lactose than the rest of the population. In fact, one study found that 24.3 percent of IBS patients had lactose malabsorption compared with just 5.7 percent of healthy subjects. Fortunately, lactose malabsorption showed a marked decrease after six weeks of diet therapy. The authors concluded that "a substantial number of IBS patients showed a clinically unrecognized lactose malabsorption, which could not be discriminated by symptoms and dietary history, and which can be treated with a lactose-restricted diet." Another study examined the impact of a lactose-restricted diet in people with IBS and lactose intolerance. The authors reported a marked improvement in symptoms with 87.5 percent of these individuals having "no complaints" in a five-year follow-up survey. This same study reported a 75 percent reduction in doctor office visits following the initiation of a lactose-restricted diet.

Since lactose intolerance can mimic IBS, it is not surprising that the two conditions can be confused by physicians. Therefore, lactose malabsorption, which is easily treatable, should be excluded as a possibility before you accept a diagnosis of irritable bowel syndrome. Overall, there are multiple studies on lactose intolerance in IBS that report "significant improvement" in 57 to 100 percent of treated cases. Moral of the story: If you have IBS, you must be tested for lactose intolerance, as these two conditions are often confused.

When evaluating IBS, many physicians will institute a lactose-free diet. Given the aforementioned studies, it is not surprising that such interventions, while not curative, are often helpful to those who suffer from IBS. Rapid small bowel transit is reported in people with IBS and lactose intolerance and may be a reason why these two conditions have overlapping symptoms.

Treating Lactose Intolerance

The best way to treat lactose intolerance is to avoid dairy products. If you're an ice-cream junkie, consider supplementing with lactase, the enzyme that digests lactose. Lactase can be purchased in most drugstores in capsules, tablets, and drops and is consumed separately from or added to milk. While lactase does not help everyone with lactase deficiency, it can make your life much easier. The lactase dosage will depend on the type of food you are eating, as dairy products have varying amounts of lactose. Some foods like "lactose-reduced" milk already have lactase added. The amount of lactase you need also depends on how lactose intolerant you are. Significant side effects have not been reported with lactase, and no drug-lactase interactions are reported. However, it is suspected that people who are lactose intolerant do not absorb calcium well. Finally, an alternative to milk is buttermilk, which has less lactose than regular milk.

Take Calcium

If you have lactose intolerance and are instructed to avoid all dairy products, make sure you supplement your diet with 1,000 to 1,500 mg of calcium daily. Of all the calcium supplements on the market, calcium citrate and calcium citrate/malate appear to have the best absorption. Since vitamin D is necessary for calcium absorption, 400 IU of vitamin D is usually taken with calcium. A daily multivitamin/mineral supplement is also recommended, since calcium competes with other minerals for absorption.

Side Effects: The most common calcium-related side effects are bloating, constipation, and gas. Other side effects include diarrhea, excessive thirst, headache, heartburn, loss of appetite, nausea, vomiting, and weakness. Rarely, kidney stones result from excessive calcium ingestion. Milk alkali syndrome is another rare side effect that occurs when people combine a dairy-rich diet with calcium carbonate supplements.

Precautions During Pregnancy: Supplementation with calcium is not recommended during pregnancy or lactation.

Drug Interactions: Interactions have been reported between calcium and albuterol, alendronate, aluminum hydroxide, barbiturates, bile acid sequestrants, caffeine, calcium channel-blockers, calcitonin, ciprofloxacin, cisplatin, corticosteroids (inhaled and oral), cycloserine, diclofenac, digoxin, digitoxin, doxycycline, erythromycin, estrogen, felodipine, gentamicin, hydroxychloroquine, indapamide, indomethacin, iron, isoniazid, itraconazole, lactase, losartan, mineral oil, minocycline, nadolol, neomycin, ofloxacin, oral contraceptives, quinidine, sodium fluoride, sodium polystyrene sulfonate, steroids, sucralfate, sulfamethoxazole, synthroid, tetracycline, thiazides, thyroid hormones, thyroxin, tobramycin, triamterene, and verapamil. If you use any of these medications, talk to your doctor before taking calcium supplements.

Special Considerations: Do not take calcium supplements without your physician's permission if you have parathyroid disease or kidney problems. Calcium should not be taken by people with bone tumors, digoxin toxicity, kidney failure, kidney stones, hyperparathyroidism, sarcoidosis, ventricular fibrillation, or a history of elevated blood levels of calcium or calcium in the urine. Also, do not take calcium if you are dehydrated, on a fluid-restricted diet, or have a history of decreased bowel motility or bowel obstruction.

SALICYLATES, AMINES, AND GLUTAMATES

Salicylates, amines, and glutamates are found naturally or added to many foods and are suspected of causing diarrhea, nausea, vomiting, abdominal pain, and excess gas. Salicylates are found in flavorings and medications, and amines are substances derived from ammonia. Glutamate is an amino acid that is used to build protein and is also found in monosodium glutamate (MSG), a common flavoring for food, which has been implicated in several sensitivity syndromes. Glutamate (glutamic acid) is found in meat, eggs, fish, and dairy products.

One meta-analysis found that foods high in salicylates and amines were frequently associated with IBS exacerbations. Given the fact that these substances are so common in foods, some authorities suspect that salicylates (and to a lesser extent, amines) may explain the food intolerances often found in IBS. If you suspect that your symptoms are related to food, try to eliminate these products from your diet for a period of one month. Given the various forms that salicylates, amines, and glutamate can take, you may consider enlisting the aid of a nutritionist to help you determine which foods you should avoid.

CAFFEINE

Caffeine is found in many foods beside coffee, including chocolate, caffeinated soft drinks, medications, and tea. If you're like many Americans, you love your coffee. Unfortunately, coffee can cause diarrhea. Caffeine is also known to cause anxiety in certain individuals, and there is evidence that people with anxiety are more sensitive to caffeine. Personally, just the thought of giving up coffee makes me anxious. Caffeine has been linked to depression as well, with reports that heavy coffee drinking can increase the risk of depression. These findings, however, are confounded by studies that indicate that long-term coffee consumption can improve mood and decrease suicide risk. While studies examining the relationship between caffeine and IBS have been inconclusive, there is some indication that IBS symptoms may be related to caffeine intake in susceptible individuals. If you find your IBS symptoms acting up after a cup of coffee, perhaps a trial caffeine separation should be attempted.

FIBER: THE PROS AND CONS

Some people with irritable bowel swear by fiber, others swear at it! We do know that fiber helps many people with IBS, especially insoluble fiber for constipation. But for some people with IBS, a high-fiber diet actually makes their symptoms worse. This is especially true for those plagued by bloating, which is often aggravated by bran-based fiber. Needless to say, dietary fiber remains one of the most controversial areas of IBS research.

America ranks among the lowest in per capita consumption of fiber worldwide. Authorities suspect that most Americans are fiber deficient given their high consumption of white flour and fruit juice. In regard to fiber, IBS treatment has to be individualized and will involve some trial and error: For some people, increasing dietary fiber will help; in others, especially those with bloating and gas, avoiding fiber may be best.

The fiber world is divided into soluble and insoluble fibers. For people with IBS, it's the insoluble fiber that is most valuable therapeutically. Insoluble fiber keeps the stool soft, thereby increasing the rate at which the stool moves through the bowel. This mechanism explains why insoluble fiber may protect against colon cancer and help people with constipation-predominate IBS.

Insoluble fiber can be found in many foods, including oatmeal, bran, whole wheat, rye, vegetables, brown rice, beans, barley, and psyllium. Beans, while rich in soluble fiber, often contain certain sugars that are difficult to absorb and are known to increase intestinal gas. Grains are also rich in insoluble fiber, whereas barley, beans, fruits, oats, psyllium, and vegetables contain both soluble and insoluble fiber.

While fiber often helps people with constipation, its role in treating diarrhea remains to be determined. While bran is reported to slow down rapid transit and accelerate slow transit, bran can exacerbate IBS in susceptible individuals. Another challenge is that the various types of fiber may affect bowel function differently.

Despite this, fiber remains a standard recommendation for both conventional and alternative healthcare practitioners, and multiple studies have documented that a high-fiber diet can help people with IBS. Fiber appears to be especially beneficial in those who suffer from constipation-predominate IBS, but approximately 25 percent of people with IBS claim that fiber exacerbates their bloating and abdominal distension. Because of this, psyllium-based compounds are often recommended, since there is evidence that psyllium is better tolerated and produces less gas in people with

IBS. Similar results are seen in carbophil agents like Citrucel and FiberCon. Multiple fiber preparations are available, and some experimentation may be needed to find the fiber supplement that works best for you.

General Recommendations: There are many different fiber supplements available. You can also increase your fiber intake by eating more fiber-rich foods. Instead of drinking fruit juice, try to gradually switch to eating whole fruits. Also, pay attention to food labels and avoid fiber-poor unbleached or white flour. If you like rice, eat wild or brown rice instead of white rice. The health benefits of eating whole-grain rice or flour products comes from the fiber-rich outer layers of these foods, which are unfortunately stripped away in the manufacturing process. Ideally, you should aim for 40 to 60 grams of fiber in your daily diet. While most fiber-containing products are rich in vitamins and minerals, fiber can interfere with the absorption of some minerals; hence, take a multivitamin/mineral supplement if you consume a high-fiber diet.

Drug Interactions: Interactions between fiber and lovastatin, propoxyphene, and verapamil have been reported. If you are using any of these medications, speak to your physician prior to supplementing your diet with fiber.

Special Considerations: Make sure you drink plenty of water when taking fiber supplements. Taking too much fiber without enough water will actually dry the stool, making constipation worse. A general rule of thumb is to drink at least 16 ounces of water per serving of fiber. With fiber, it's important to start with a low dose and work your way up gradually to a maintenance dose. Consult your doctor if you have a history of bowel obstruction, severe constipation, or scleroderma before taking a fiber supplement or beginning a fiber-rich diet; there are reports of fiber exacerbating constipation or causing dangerous bowel obstruction in these individuals.

Wheat Bran

Wheat has been cultivated for at least 10,000 years. The bran comes from the milling of wheat. It contains about 20 percent indigestible cellulose, which is also the foundation of vegetable fiber and one of the most common polysaccharides. Indigestible cellulose helps increase stool bulk, making it easier to pass. Wheat is used in many food products including flour, bread, cereal, and farina. The bran found in the outer layer of the grain holds the most potential for gastrointestinal disorders.

Carbophil—An Alternative to Bran

If you can't tolerate bran, consider carbophil, a non-laxative hydrophilic colloid (calcium polycarbophil) that absorbs water and increases the bulk and water content of the stool while keeping the stool from becoming too liquid. Carbophil agents are reported to produce less gas than traditional bran and are the fiber supplement of choice for many people with IBS, constipation, and diarrhea. Common polycarbophil compounds include Citrucel, FiberCon, Equalactin, and Mitrolan. Studies have found that carbophil produces significant differences in bowel complaints (constipation, alternating diarrhea/constipation, nausea, pain, and bloating.

Dose: Typical dosage of carbophil is 500 milligrams two to four times daily; must be taken with at least 8 ounces of water.

Side Effects: abdominal pain, bloating, diarrhea, nausea, trouble swallowing, and vomiting.

Contraindications: Do not use this product if you have a history of bowel obstruction, recent abdominal surgery, active inflammatory bowel disease (Crohn's disease or ulcerative colitis), a sudden change in bowel habits over the past two weeks, or during bouts of active abdominal pain, nausea, or vomiting.

Drug Interactions: Interactions between carbophil and tetracycline have been reported, so speak to your doctor if you are using this medication before taking carbophil.

Special Considerations: Make sure you drink at least 8 ounces of liquid with each dose. Results are usually seen in two to three days. Laxative and laxative-like products should not be used for more than a week without a physician's supervision. If you experience trouble breathing, chest pain, difficulty swallowing, or vomiting after using this product, contact your doctor immediately or call 911, as these symptoms may indicate that the product is potentially blocking your esophagus or airway.

For people with IBS who want to increase their fiber, the whole grain packs the most punch, but some people are allergic to wheat, and this can result in a variety of symptoms, from bloating to eczema. Celiac disease is a common bowel disorder characterized by a gluten intolerance (gluten is commonly found in wheat, barley, and rye). So, the whole grain may not be an option for some people with IBS.

Bran, however, has a mixed reputation in IBS, with some people failing to improve or maintain a positive response. Conversely, many people, especially those with constipation, are genuinely helped by bran. In many people with IBS, bran causes increased pain and bloating, a finding supported by clinical trials and by numerous patient accounts that blame bran for worsening their symptoms. One study found that in people with IBS who had moderate to severe bloating, their small bowel transit time was significantly faster compared to people without IBS. The researchers discovered that in those without IBS, bran accelerates transit time and colon clearance without causing symptoms. But bowel transit time is already rapid in IBS patients with bloating and can't be further accelerated by bran, which nevertheless aggravated their pain and bloating. For those with IBS whose bloating and pain are worsened by bran, it may be the result of a rapid filling of the ascending colon, which then fails to respond to the bran with accelerated clearing. Bran ingestion would simply make the situation worse by adding bulk and causing gas from fermentation.

Another study examined wheat bran in thirty-eight people with IBS who had not previously undergone bran treatment. Constipation "improved significantly" with bran (a result not seen with placebo), with increased stool weight. Forty-seven percent believed that their symptoms had improved with bran, while 53 percent felt their symptoms remained unchanged or got worse. Unfortunately, diarrhea was not improved and made worse with bran (however, other studies have reported that bran can help people with IBS-related diarrhea). There was significant improvement in all symptoms except diarrhea, distension, flatulence, and heartburn during treatment with bran, but similar findings were reported for the placebo group. Pain and urgency were actually exacerbated by bran. In the final analysis, constipation was the only symptom that improved significantly on bran.

One controlled trial examined wheat bran in twenty-six people with IBS who consumed either a high- or low-fiber diet of unprocessed wheat bran for six weeks. After six weeks, those on a high-fiber diet showed significant improvement in symptoms and a reduction in colonic motor activity. Specifically, the frequency of pain was reduced in patients on the high-fiber diet, and seven patients reported improved bowel habits. None of the high-fiber group reported a worsening in bowel habits. The frequency of bowel actions increased slightly in the high-fiber group, and the passage of mucus decreased. The researchers concluded that patients with IBS should increase their daily intake of wheat fiber, as their investigation demonstrated significant benefits from a diet high in wheat bran. They also agreed that individualization of treatment was probably best for IBS, by tailoring the diet and the dose of bran to the preferences of each patient.

General Recommendations: Why some people respond to bran and others don't remains a subject of active investigation, but some authorities suspect a wheat sensitivity may be to blame. (Brown rice, oatmeal, and vegetables are less likely to exacerbate IBS symptoms in people who are sensitive to wheat bran.) The questions surrounding the use of bran in IBS are likely to receive intense scrutiny for years to come. What should you do? It's fair to say that if you have constipation-predominant IBS, bran may be worth a trial. For those with diarrhea, bloating, or pain, the jury is still out regarding bran, calcium and further research is needed.

I recommend a trial of bran for every person with IBS. While what works for one person may not work for the next, at the very worst your symptoms will temporarily flare and you'll throw the bran in the garbage. At best, you'll discover that bran helps your symptoms and develop a happy and healthy relationship with it.

Dose: Miller's bran is frequently used, with a typical dose of 2 tablespoons four times a day, for a total of 12 to 16 grams daily. As many people find the flavor of bran supplements unappealing, try to increase the bran content of your diet using bran-rich foods such as whole-wheat bread, brown rice, or bran-based breakfast cereals.

Drug Interactions: Interactions between bran and lovastatin, propoxyphene, and verapamil have been reported. If you are using any of these medications, speak to your physician prior to supplementing your diet with bran.

Special Considerations: Make sure you drink plenty of water when taking bran. Too much bran without enough water will dry the stool, making constipation worse. Drink at least 16 ounces of water per serving of bran. Consult your doctor if you have a history of bowel obstruction, severe constipation, or scleroderma before taking bran. Bran is also known to reduce calcium absorption so consider taking a calcium supplement. This is especially true for men and women who want to help prevent osteoporosis. See the discussion of calcium on page 80.

Barley and Rye

Rye is a grass that can survive in harsh climates, making it a particularly important dietary staple. Like wheat, rye is used in the production of many foods such as cereals, baked goods, flour, and bread. A great source of fiber, rye may cause fewer problems for people with IBS who are sensitive to wheat bran.

Barley is the most ancient of grains, dating back to the Stone Age. Like rye, barley can be grown just about anywhere and is an excellent source of fiber, often better tolerated by people with IBS who are sensitive to wheat bran. Barley is a rarity in commercially prepared foods, as it is used mostly for making beer and animal feed. Scotch barley (whole barley) contains the most bran, and, like all grains, barley comes in flour, flake, and other forms. The beta-glucan found in barley is suspected to lower cholesterol by binding and helping to eliminate cholesterol-rich bile acids. Conversely, barley may play a role in food allergies and is frequently eliminated in hypoallergenic diets.

Barley and rye can be purchased in most stores.

Special Considerations: Make sure you store barley and rye in sealed plastic or glass containers in a cool, dry place, as the oils can spoil if exposed to air, moisture, or sunlight. Barley takes more time to cook, so for quicker results, soak overnight. Since rye and barley contain gluten, they should be avoided by people with celiac disease.

Psyllium (Flea Seed, Ispaghula, Spogel, *Plantago ovata, Plantago ispaghula)*

Native to India and Iran, psyllium has been used to treat diabetes, high cholesterol, and several gastrointestinal complaints, including constipation and irritable bowel. Psyllium husk is often better tolerated in people with IBS who are sensitive to wheat bran. Rich in fiber and mucilage, psyllium is a natural bulk-forming laxative. Psyllium is frequently used in over-the-counter remedies to treat constipation because of its water-hungry husk that expands when hydrated. Psyllium is a hydrophilic colloid, meaning it absorbs water and increases stool bulk, helping to keep the stool hydrated and easier to pass. Furthermore, by increasing stool bulk, psyllium helps trigger the bowel reflex needed for successful defecation. Psyllium also helps keep the stool from becoming too liquid and is used in IBS for both constipation and diarrhea. Psyllium is reported to produce less gas than traditional fiber and is the fiber supplement of choice for many people with IBS.

Multiple studies have examined ispaghula husk for IBS and demonstrated that it can improve the overall sense of well-being as well as help relieve IBS-related symptoms. One trial examined the impact of two pharmaceuticals, lorazepam and hyoscine butylbromide, along with ispaghula husk in various combinations and against placebo. The authors found that only with ispaghula was the patient improvement between the real and placebo preparation "statistically significant." A similar study found that ispaghula was significantly more effective than bran.

Another placebo-controlled trial in twenty people with IBS reported that ispaghula husks resulted in improvement in overall symptoms and in satisfying bowel movements, but did not influence abdominal pain and flatulence. A small number of subjects experienced a change in bowel transit time, but these changes were not considered significant. The enhanced bowel satisfaction was probably due to increased stool weight caused by ispaghula.

One study compared psyllium to wheat bran in thirty IBS patients for six weeks. There was improvement in stool frequency in both groups, but the effect of psyllium seeds exceeded that of wheat bran. Psyllium improved abdominal pain more than bran, and abdominal distension was exacerbated by wheat bran, but it decreased with psyllium. The authors concluded that psyllium seeds were superior to wheat bran in treating stool frequency and abdominal distension, and it should be recommended over bran for IBS and constipation.

Finally, one double-blind, placebo-controlled study from England found that ispaghula decreased transit time significantly, especially in patients with initially high transit times, a common feature of IBS. Ispaghula also reduced the number of days without a bowel movement, an especially important measure for people with constipation. Ispaghula significantly increased overall well-being in patients with IBS and improved bowel habits and transit time in those with constipation.

While psyllium and other fiber-rich agents are normally used for constipation, there is evidence that psyllium may also help people with diarrhea. One trial found that 9 to 30 grams of psyllium seed helped people with diarrhea by making the stool less loose. While this study did not specifically examine individuals with IBS, the results are encouraging and demonstrate that psyllium may help those with diarrhea-predominant IBS. Given the results of these multiple studies, a trial of psyllium is clearly indicated if you have constipation-predominant IBS.

Dose: Most authorities recommend 5 grams (1 teaspoon) of psyllium husks three times a day. If you use whole seeds, 10 to 30 grams (2 to 6 teaspoons) is usually recommended, divided between three equal doses. Psyllium should be taken with meals to ensure that it will be integrated into the stool. Common psyllium-containing compounds include Konsyl, Metamucil, and L.A. Formula.

Side Effects: Side effects from psyllium-containing compounds are uncommon but may include indigestion and bloating. While there are some individuals whose IBS gets worse with psyllium, it is suspected that these people are intolerant of insoluble fiber and may be better off using soluble forms of fiber, such as whole fruit.

Drug Interactions: Interactions between psyllium and lithium and mesalamine have been reported. If you are taking either of these medications, speak to your doctor before supplementing with psyllium.

Special Considerations: Make sure you drink 16 ounces of water with each serving, since psyllium works by absorbing water. Also, remember to drink psyllium immediately after mixing with water or else it will quickly thicken. Do not use psyllium if you have poorly controlled diabetes or a history of bowel obstruction.

Partially Hydrolyzed Guar Gum

Partially hydrolyzed guar gum (PHGG), a fiber-like product, is a newcomer to the IBS medicine cabinet, with the first study examining this agent published in 2002. Researchers evaluated 188 people with IBS for twelve weeks, comparing PHGG (5 grams daily) to wheat bran (30 grams daily). The study group consisted of individuals with diarrhea, constipation, and alternating diarrhea-constipation IBS. Both bran and PHGG improved pain and bowel habits, but people who used PHGG reported greater subjective improvement than those in the bran group. After four weeks, the patients were allowed to switch treatments: 49.9 percent converted from fiber to PHGG, but only 10.9 percent switched from PHGG to fiber, indicating a strong preference for PHGG. While this is the first study evaluating PHGG, initial results are encouraging. PHGG was better tolerated and preferred by patients, meaning a higher probability of success than bran and making it a good choice for fiber supplementation.

Dose: The typical dose of PHGG is 5 grams daily.

NOT ALL FATS ARE CREATED EQUAL

Who doesn't like fat? Fat makes food taste great, and eating *lots* of fat probably conferred a survival advantage in our prehistoric ancestors. This should not be surprising since, pound for pound, fat packs the most energy per unit consumed. These days, however, we no longer need to hunt for food or flee from hostile tribes, so all that fat goes to places it doesn't belong—thighs, bellies, and arteries.

Not all fats, however, are created equal. Polyunsaturated fatty acids, omega-3 and omega-6, are "good" fats. What should be avoided are the saturated fats commonly found in baked goods, such as donuts and potato chips. Also avoid margarine and hydrogenated oils—these products are loaded with artery-clogging trans-fatty acids, a type of saturated fat that is far worse for your heart than butter. These trans-fatty acids wreak havoc with the normal metabolism of heart-friendly omega-3s and omega-6s, the good guys.

In some people with IBS, enhanced bowel contractions have been found following the ingestion of a high-fat meal.

When I cook, in addition to using my favorite heart-friendly oil, I use wine. Wine adds flavor and helps keep food from burning, thereby allowing you to use less butter and oil. Healthy omega-3 and omega-6 oils include canola, flaxseed, hemp, and walnut oil. Try to maintain a balance between omega-3s and omega-6s by using a different cooking oil each time you cook.

Omega-3 and Omega-6 Fatty Acids

Fish is considered part of a healthy diet because it contains essential fatty acids (fish oils), such as alpha-linolenic acid (omega-3) and linoleic acid (omega-6). These fats are "essential" because our bodies can't make them,

The BRAT Diet

BRAT stands for bananas, rice, apples, and toast—foods that are rich in fiber and potassium and recommended by some physicians during bouts of acute diarrhea. At the present time, there are no studies evaluating the BRAT diet for IBS. Nevertheless, this diet is fiber-rich and can offer benefits to IBS sufferers who regularly have diarrhea.

and we have to rely on dietary sources. Fish oils are also heart-friendly, helping to lower triglycerides and keep atherosclerosis in check. Because of their anti-inflammatory properties, fish oils are also used to treat a number of conditions, including high blood pressure, diabetes, and schizophrenia.

The chief omega-3 acids are eicosapentaenoic acid (EPA) and docosahexaenoic acid (DHA), which can be found in a variety of fish, including anchovies, albacore tuna, herring, sardines, and salmon. You can even find omega-3s in flaxseed oil, walnut oil, and game meat. Or try grandma's old favorite, cod liver oil. While omega-6 is a good fat, too much may increase your risk of heart disease and high blood pressure. Nevertheless, I strongly recommend that you maintain a healthy balance between the two omegas, since these fats are essential, and your body must have them.

As we learned in Chapter 4, researchers found that if you treat IBS like you would treat depression, people often get better regardless of whether or not they were depressed. Several disorders of fatty acid metabolism have been described in depression, including low omega-3 levels. One study found that the concentration of omega-3s was lower in the red cell membranes of depressed patients, and that the lower the omega-3 level, the more severe the depression. Furthermore, too much omega-6 can increase the risk of depression (in some depressed patients with low omega-3s, there is a "compensatory" increase in omega-6s). Conversely, there is evidence that people who consume high levels of omega-3s have lower rates of depression. It is theorized that fatty acids and antidepressant drugs like lithium work on common pathways.

While there is no direct evidence that fish oils can help IBS, this should not dissuade people from increasing the amount of healthy fish in their diet. Considering the important role fish oils play in preserving overall health and our new knowledge regarding the Brain-Gut Model and depression, eating fish is a win-win situation.

Dose: Most authorities recommend approximately 10 grams of fish oil daily. You can meet these requirements simply by mixing a tablespoon of flaxseed oil with your favorite food daily. Always remember to maintain a healthy balance between omega-3s and omega-6s to avoid increasing your risk of heart disease. Nutritional experts also recommend taking your fish oil with an antioxidant such as vitamin E to preserve the potency of these oils, which are extremely sensitive to oxygen degradation.

Side Effects: Side effects are uncommon, but can include stomach upset. (This can be avoided by taking "enteric-coated" supplements.) Since fish oil can rarely raise LDL cholesterol, people with heart disease or high cholesterol should talk to their doctor before taking supplements. The same is true for individuals with diabetes, as fish oil can potentially raise blood sugar. There is limited evidence that these undesirable effects on blood sugar can be prevented by taking vitamin E or by regular exercise (three times a week).

Drug Interactions: Fish and cod liver oil can react with cyclosporine, pravastatin, and simvastatin, so it's a good idea to check with your doctor before supplementing if you are taking these medications. Finally, consult a doctor if you are pregnant or intend to regularly take cod liver oil that contains more than 25,000 IU of vitamin A or 800 IU of vitamin D.

Chapter 6

Vitamin, Mineral, and Herbal Supplements

When I started writing about integrative medicine several years ago, I was skeptical about vitamins, minerals, and herbs, along with any therapy that didn't involve high technology or at least a powerful pharmaceutical. As I researched various alternative therapies, it dawned on me that many of them really worked. I was pleasantly surprised to learn that the people who researched alternative therapies came from similar backgrounds to mine and experienced the same difficulties every scientist faces when seeking the truth. It has been a profound learning experience that has forever changed the way I look at health and medicine. So, before we delve into the subject of supplements for irritable bowel syndrome, let us briefly examine the challenges and problems that scientists face when conducting research.

SCIENTIFIC RESEARCH AND SCIENTIFIC UNCERTAINTY

Some say that every particle of matter has an opposite, a piece of antimatter. The same can be said for many scientific studies: for every study that says X is true, there is another study that says Y is true, and X is either wrong or was not as important as everyone thought. Controversy in science is good and keeps the research interesting, presenting new challenges that force our knowledge to grow. The public, however, as a rule is uneasy with the concept that for doctors and scientists, uncertainty is a fact of scientific life.

Another important lesson is that no study is perfect. Any decent epidemiologist or statistician can find a flaw in almost any study. Many times researchers must make difficult decisions that can strengthen one part of a study at the expense of another. One problem we commonly see in nutritional supplement research is that many early studies attempted to investigate the short-term effects of supplementation, an approach that often yields discouraging results. Not surprising since we now understand that diet and supplements achieve their greatest benefit over months or years, not just a few days.

Now, don't get me wrong, physicians do know a lot about the human body. We also know about IBS and how to treat it. Few doctors would deny that altered bowel motility and IBS are linked. Controversy rages, however, over the true impact emotions have on IBS. So, while there are many things about IBS that physicians agree on, there are also many unresolved questions that at present are subject to intense debate.

We also have to understand that scientists and physicians are trained to remain skeptical, to never accept anything at face value. It's not good enough for one study to report that fiber helps people with IBS. The "scientific method" demands that additional studies be performed to see if similar results can be achieved, a quality known as reproducibility. Reproducibility is central to the scientific method and is a major reason why controversy exists in medicine. It is also the reason why it often takes years for a particular finding to be accepted by the scientific community. Reproducibility is so important that, without it, as far as the scientific method is concerned, there can be no facts.

Scientific discovery is not like a movie, with the wild-haired scientist surrounded by test tubes suddenly shouting, "Eureka!" Finding the truth is hard work and normally involves years of research coupled with persistent controversy. How we get to know what we know can be divided into three general stages: hypothesis, research-publication-controversy, and acceptance-rejection. This process of discovery can last for decades, but it is the only way we can be remotely certain about the accuracy of scientific research.

What usually happens first is that someone reports an expected or unexpected finding during a study. From this new finding, a hypothesis is generated. For instance, a group of researchers study the relationship between diet and health and find that people with IBS whose diets are rich in fiber have fewer symptoms. Another scientist reads their report and says to herself, "That's interesting. I wonder if giving extra fiber will reduce their symptoms." This is the hypothesis: Fiber supplementation can reduce IBS severity.

The researcher then designs a study to test her hypothesis. She develops a randomly controlled, double-blind study by taking a group of people with IBS and giving half the participants fiber pills and the other half a placebo. She then follows these two groups for a period of time, during which she measures a variety of IBS-related variables, such as abdominal pain and quality of life scores. Once the study is completed, the test results are compared between the two groups and are presented to the scientific community, usually by being published in a scientific journal.

Other scientists see her report and decide to reproduce those results to determine if they're valid. This is where things get complicated. How a study is designed depends on the researcher and the type of data being collected. There are several basic study designs, each with their own strengths and weaknesses, and no two studies are exactly alike. What evolves from these efforts is that multiple studies examining the relationship between fiber and IBS begin to appear in the scientific literature. What often happens in early research is that some studies say fiber helps, some say fiber doesn't help, and other studies are inconclusive. Researchers then critically review the published studies for flaws and design improved studies that they hope will yield reproducible results, a process that can take years to decades. This cycle of publication followed by critical review and additional publications is called the research-publication-controversy stage.

Ideally, over a period of years, what you find is a gradually evolving body of literature with more consistent findings. Once this occurs, we are at the acceptance-rejection part of the process. Yet, no matter how consistent the findings are among a group of papers, it is not uncommon to see newly published work that contradicts the established consensus. Sometimes these contradictory studies simply result from design flaws and are quickly dismissed. Other times, such studies represent the first step in toppling a medical dogma.

THE CHALLENGES OF NUTRITIONAL RESEARCH

Vitamin deficiencies usually occur in one of three ways in humans: inadequate intake, improper absorption, or increased demand. In people with IBS, it appears that inadequate intake and absorption play the most important roles in their deficiencies. One of the problems with supplement research is that if an individual is deficient in substance A, chances are he or she is also deficient in substances X, Y, and Z. In other words, vitamin and mineral deficiencies do not occur in a vacuum, as the dietary or medical derangements that created the original deficiency usually cause other deficiencies. This is why it is difficult to study one particular deficiency without taking into consideration others. Further complicating the picture, proper bowel function rests not on a single nutrient but on an entire symphony of vitamins and minerals that are responsible for overall health, including bowel health. This is why it is difficult to test the impact of supplementing a particular vitamin or mineral on IBS.

About forty years ago, scientists began to pay serious attention to diet and its impact on health, investigating this relationship both retrospectively and prospectively. Retrospective means that you search data you already have for a particular relationship. The best studies, however, are usually prospective, which means you collect new data and then examine it for a relationship.

Over the past twenty years, we have witnessed an explosion of publications that link diet and emotions to IBS. This does not mean that every case of IBS can be blamed on diet or psychological factors. This simply means that the scientific community recognizes that diet and emotions play roles in IBS. The relationship between IBS and dietary supplements remains a topic of ongoing debate.

Scientists face a number of challenges and problems when conducting research. As you read this chapter, you will notice that most researchers report that a particular supplement benefited some but not all study participants. For example, in a study examining the effect of supplement X on IBS, the authors may report that only 54 percent of the participants had a favorable response to supplementation. This is a common finding because the medical condition we call "IBS" is the shared endpoint of multiple abnormal biological pathways. Many roads lead to IBS, and every person with IBS has a unique set of genetic, environmental, and psychological influences that result in the expression of these pathways. These unique pathways are the reason why we have multiple types of IBS that often respond to different treatment.

These multiple pathways present a special challenge to researchers still in the process of understanding how they work and interact. IBS probably results from a complex interplay between genes and environment, and this is why we see a particular supplement work for some, but not for all, people. Even though many roads lead to IBS, they tend to end at the same place. The most successful therapies target these common pathways.

Nutrient researchers also have to contend with different diets among study subjects. The ideal supplement study would examine two groups of people with identical medical conditions, nutrient deficiencies, and diets while comparing the effect of supplementation versus no supplementation. Though we can find people with similar medical conditions, it's difficult to control and monitor individual diets. With animal studies, you can totally control an animal's diet and the integrity of the study data. The tough part about human diet studies is that people cheat. While scientists have mathematical models that correct data for different diets, dietary aberrations will always remain a potential source of error.

While the concept that diet impacts on health is generally accepted, we remain in the research-publication-controversy stage when it comes to individual supplements for IBS. Some supplements, like psyllium, have accumulated a substantial body of literature supporting their use. For other supplements, research is intense and findings hotly debated.

EVIDENCE-BASED MEDICINE

Doctors use many therapies because they work, not because there are multiple scientific studies documenting that a particular treatment is superior to another. We are all, in part, a product of our history, and modern medicine is no exception. Mercifully, physicians also learn from their mistakes, and when a treatment does more harm than good, it is quickly abandoned. Over the past decade, physicians have begun to realize that choosing a therapy just because that's the way they have always treated a condition is not good enough. These concerns have resulted in a revolution called "evidence-based medicine" (EBM), a relatively new and exciting chapter in medical history. EBM demands that therapies make scientific sense and are rigorously tested to see if they actually offer benefit.

One of the fundamental tenets of EBM is that the best way to test if a treatment works is to take a group of people with medical condition X and randomly divide them into treatment group A and placebo group B, with neither doctor nor patient knowing who is in each group, and then see how they do. This basic technique is called a double-blind, randomized, controlled trial (RCT) and is the preferred evidence-based research design. With RCTs, the larger the population, the more you can generalize the results. This is not to say that small study groups make a bad trial; it only means that, in general, the more participants the better.

There is one more study design you should know about—the meta-analysis. Meta-analysis is considered one of the most powerful EBM tools. While RCTs examine individual groups of patients, meta-analysis examines the validity of multiple RCTs. Put another way, meta-analysis critically analyzes a group of RCTs, examining them for the quality of their design and then offering a summary of their pooled conclusions.

With respect to IBS research, results are usually reported as subjective and objective findings. Objective findings are variables that can be measured using standardized instruments and are therefore reproducible. Typical objective findings in IBS research include number of bowel movements and bowel transit times. Subjective findings are usually reported in IBS research as "quality of life" scores, calculated from a standardized survey.

As a rule, scientists prefer objective findings to subjective findings. Most people with IBS, however, care more about how well they feel. In the end, subjective and objective findings are equally important. While it is vital to measure objective improvement in bowel function, the most important therapy variable for the people suffering from IBS is "Do I feel better?"

SUPPLEMENTATION 101

As with any emerging field of medicine, controversy exists over the true impact supplements have on IBS. There are many beneficial supplements, and you may wonder how to choose the supplements that are right for you. Nobody wants to be popping fifty pills a day, so this chapter will help you make smart supplement choices.

Start by taking two standard supplements that will not only help your IBS but will also protect you against other diseases for which you might be at risk. After two months, if your bowels do not improve, continue taking your two standard supplements and experiment with additional individual supplements for your IBS. Give each supplement a four-week trial while recording symptoms in your IBS diary. I also suggest you get tested for vitamin and mineral deficiencies and, with the aid of a skilled healthcare professional, correct any deficiency found.

If you decide to take an individual supplement, carefully review with a physician or a pharmacist all the prescription and nonprescription products you are using. While most vitamin and mineral supplements are safe when used as directed, the potential for drug interactions is best avoided. If you can't decide which supplement is right for you, I suggest enlisting the aid of a trusted healthcare professional who can help you decide.

Remember that nutritional supplements are only a small part of the IBS treatment picture. The purpose of this book is to eliminate or markedly improve your IBS. The foundation of good health and proper bowel function rests not with supplements alone; rather, a healthy life demands dealing with psychological issues, practicing good nutrition, and getting regular exercise. Supplements can certainly help IBS, but they are only one piece of the complex puzzle of health. Do not be lulled into believing that a pill is going to solve your problems. Supplements can certainly play an important role in IBS, but they must be incorporated into a larger plan of healthy living that protects the entire body.

CARAWAY OIL

Native to Africa, Asia, and Europe, the seeds and fruit of caraway have been used since 1500 B.C. when the Egyptians used it to aid digestion and relieve gas. Shakespeare makes reference to caraway as a digestive aid for Falstaff in *Henry IV.* Modern herbalists use caraway for IBS, indigestion, and gingivitis. Caraway is a carminative (relieves gas) that contains the volatile oils carvone and limonene. These oils may also reduce bowel spasm. Caraway oil for IBS has been extensively studied, and Germany's Commission E made a positive risk-benefit analysis for this herb in dyspepsia.

Caraway oil is reported to have spasmolytic and antibacterial activity that can help relieve IBS symptoms. It is usually combined with other carminative herbs, such as peppermint and fennel. One German prospective, randomized, double-blind trial examined the effect of a preparation of caraway and peppermint oils in 223 people with IBS. The study demonstrated a statistically significant decline in pain intensity and abdominal pain frequency. The side effect profile was low for the combined oil preparation. While more studies are needed, initial studies on caraway oil are encouraging, so a trial of this herb is worthy of consideration for people with IBS.

Dose: The most common dosage of caraway oil is 0.05 to 0.2 milliliters of enteric-coated volatile oil three times a day, usually taken with another carminative.

Side Effects: Side effects are rare; however, caraway oil should not be used by children under two years of age. Excessive dosages may induce abortions in pregnant women and can cause nervous system problems.

Drug Interactions: None have been identified.

FOLIC ACID (FOLATE, FOLINIC ACID, AND METHYFOLATE)

Folic acid is involved in DNA and RNA synthesis, playing a vital role in cellular reproduction and growth, and it also helps reduce homocysteine (important for heart health). Folic acid deficiency may play a role in IBS, depression, and sugar intolerance. There is evidence that people with IBS have inadequate intakes of many nutrients, including folic acid. Low blood folic acid concentrations have also been associated with fructose malabsorption. This is relevant because sugar intolerance may be partially or totally responsible for some IBS symptoms in select individuals.

Researchers have found that depression may be linked to folic acid deficiency, and supplements may potentiate the therapeutic effect of antidepressants as well as make people feel better. One double-blind, controlled trial examined the effect of 200 micrograms of folic acid in seventy-five patients on lithium, a medication commonly used to treat mental disorders. According to the study, those with the highest blood concentrations of folate showed a significant reduction in the affective morbidity. If you are depressed, make sure to check for a folic acid deficiency.

Dietary Sources: Beans, brewer's yeast, grain products (flour, rice), lentils, meat, orange juice, spinach, and green leafy veggies.

Dose: Folic acid deficiency is often treated with high-dose folic acid, which should only be used under a doctor's supervision. Most authorities typically recommend 100 to 400 micrograms of folic acid daily.

Side Effects: No significant side effects have been reported. Rare side effects include bronchospasm, itching, and rash.

Precautions During Pregnancy: Folic acid supplements are safe and encouraged during pregnancy to help prevent birth defects. Talk to your doctor about the right dose for you.

Drug Interactions: Interactions are reported with antacids, antiseizure medications, aspirin, barbiturates, bile acid sequestrants, cancer chemotherapy, colestipol, cycloserine, diuretics, erythromycin, famotidine, fluoxetine, indomethacin, isoniazid, lithium, medroxyprogesterone, metformin, methotrexate, neomycin, nitrous oxide, nizatidine, oral contraceptives, phenytoin, piroxicam, pyrimethamine, salsalate, sulfamethoxazole, sulindac, tetracycline, triamterene, and trimethoprim/ sulfamethoxazole. If you are using any of these medications, check with your physician before taking folic acid.

Special Considerations: Folic acid supplementation can delay the diagnosis of vitamin B_{12} deficiency. If you have a history of anemia, speak to your doctor before taking folic acid.

GRAPEFRUIT SEED EXTRACT (GSE)

Grapefruit seed extract may be effective in reducing some symptoms of irritable bowel. In one study on GSE in twenty-five people with IBS, individuals were treated with GSE (either 2 drops of a 0.5 percent solution twice daily or 150 milligrams of extract in a capsule three times daily). After four weeks, participants reported decreased abdominal pain, gas, and constipation. (The encapsulated form was most effective.)

Dose: While GSE is available in liquid and capsule form, it appears that the encapsulated form is most effective in IBS. The usual dosage is one capsule (100 to 200 milligrams) of dried extract taken two to three times daily.

Side Effects: No significant side effects or drug interactions have been reported with GSE.

IBEROGAST (STW-5)

Hailing from Germany, Iberogast is an herbal combination containing bitter candy tuft, lemon balm leaves, angelica root, celandine herbs, milk thistle fruit, chamomile flower, peppermint leaves, caraway fruit, and licorice root extracts. (STW-5-S is the cousin of Iberogast that does not contain bitter candy fruit because it may have an additive effect on dyspeptic symptoms.) In one randomly controlled trial, sixty patients with functional dyspepsia were treated with Iberogast, STW-5-S, or placebo for four weeks. According to the study, both herbal preparations showed a clinically significant improvement of gastrointestinal symptoms. The researchers did not observe any "statistically significant" differences between Iberogast and STW-5-S.

Dose: The usual dose of Iberogast is 20 drops, three times daily.

Side Effects: No significant side effects or drug-herb interactions have been reported with Iberogast.

PEPPERMINT OIL

Peppermint is actually a hybrid of spearmint and water mint that was first grown in England in the 1700s. Besides being used extensively in IBS, peppermint has also been used in the treatment of upset stomach, colic, tension headaches, and gingivitis. The active ingredients of peppermint are menthol and menthone, which act as carminatives and inhibit gas formation. Peppermint is also thought to have antispasmodic activity, relaxing gastrointestinal smooth muscle by reducing calcium influx. As you may recall, colonic spasm is one of the mechanisms behind IBS symptoms. It is also reported that peppermint oil has antimicrobial action, which may play a role in fighting IBS. While peppermint oil has been used alone to treat

IBS, emerging evidence suggests that peppermint/caraway oil combinations offer superior results. Peppermint oil for IBS has been extensively studied, and Germany's Commission E has made a positive risk-benefit analysis for using this herb for dyspepsia.

Several studies have found that enteric-coated peppermint oil helps relieve IBS pain. One prospective, randomized, double-blind, placebo-controlled trial examined 110 individuals with IBS who took one enteric-coated peppermint oil capsule three to four times daily for one month. According to the study, 79 percent experienced an alleviation of abdominal pain with twenty-nine subjects being pain free. Additionally, 83 percent reported less abdominal distension, 83 percent had reduced stool frequency, 73 percent had less intestinal rumbling, and 79 percent reported less flatulence. This study did not, however, report any impact on nausea, acid regurgitation, belching, and heartburn. Side effects were rare and included heartburn and skin rash. The low side effect profile was attributed to the enteric-coating that delays peppermint oil release. Another double-blind study found that patients felt significantly better while taking peppermint oil, particularly in relieving abdominal symptoms.

A peppermint and caraway oil combination called Enteroplant has also proven effective. Enteroplant, which contains 90 milligrams of peppermint oil and 50 milligrams of caraway oil in an enteric-coated capsule, was recently studied in a double-blind, placebo-controlled trial in forty-five patients. According to the authors, statistically significant results were obtained after four weeks of treatment, with 63.2 percent of the treatment group free from abdominal pain and 94.5 percent experiencing an improvement in their overall symptom score. Additionally, 89.5 percent reported decreased pain intensity. Reductions in "feelings of pressure, weight, tension and fullness, eructation, and flatulence" were also reported. The herbal combination was "excellently tolerated," with the success being attributed to the synergistic effect of the peppermint and caraway oils. It was thought that a normalization of motility due to a reduction in spasms contributed to the reduced pain. These findings offer a strong endorsement for peppermint and caraway oil combinations in the treatment of IBS.

Dose: One to two enteric-coated tablets taken two to three times daily is the usual dose. Teas and peppermint leaf tablets are also available; however, enteric-coated tablets are preferred for IBS. The typical dosage of Enteroplant is one capsule three times daily.

Side Effects: Upset stomach, esophageal reflux, and stomach/rectal burning are reported with peppermint oil. These side effects can often be avoided by using an enteric-coated preparation. Rectal burning is caused by unabsorbed methanol in the stool. Side effects with Enteroplant are uncommon, but include belching, nausea, flatulence, and rare gastric irritation.

Drug Interactions: Interactions with peppermint oil and cisapride, a drug whose use has been discontinued, have been reported. If you are using this medication, speak to your doctor before taking peppermint oil.

Special Considerations: Talk to your pediatrician before using peppermint oil in children or infants. Do not use peppermint oil without your physician's permission if you have liver disease, chronic heartburn, gallbladder disease or gallstones, or a history of bile duct obstruction.

VITAMIN A (RETINOL)

Vitamin A is needed to turn light into signals that the brain can recognize so we can see, so retinol deficiency results in night blindness. Vitamin A also keeps epithelial cell membranes intact. Besides helping to protect against infection, vitamin A can stimulate immune function. Vitamin A also helps cells grow normally: Since a fundamental cancer mechanism is deranged cellular maturation, vitamin A can protect against a variety of cancers. Vitamin A is also used to treat night blindness, measles, acne, and celiac disease.

Vitamin A supplements are important for IBS-associated diarrhea, which can lead to malabsorption-induced vitamin A deficiency. Even if you don't have a genuine vitamin A deficiency, consider taking a vitamin A supplement as people with IBS have inadequate intakes of many nutrients, including vitamin A.

Dietary Sources: Fruit, meat, milk, liver, poultry, vegetables, dairy products, and cod liver oil. Beta-carotene, a powerful antioxidant found in vegetables and fruits, can be converted to vitamin A by the body.

Dose: While vitamin A is dosed as high as 100,000 IU a day for lung infections and measles, high-dose supplements are used only for short periods of time, one to three days. Most authorities recommend 10,000 to 25,000 IU of vitamin A daily for long-term supplementation. Since only a small percentage of beta-carotene is converted to vitamin A, beta-carotene supplements should not result in retinol toxicity. Vitamin A is best absorbed when taken with food.

Probiotics

The bowel normally contains bacteria, such as *Lactobacilli*, that perform vital functions such as preventing the overgrowth of potentially harmful bacteria. In some individuals, IBS may be caused by alterations in intestinal microflora, as some normal bowel microorganisms produce excess gas, which may partially explain the increased gas and abdominal pain seen in IBS. Probiotics (supplements of these "friendly" bacteria) are often used in alternative medicine for the treatment of infectious and antibiotic-associated diarrhea. Probiotic therapy attempts to alter the bowel's microflora population in IBS.

One study found that 78 percent of IBS patients had bacterial overgrowth, which was subsequently treated with antibiotics. According to the researchers, those who successfully eradicated their bacterial overgrowth showed an improvement in irritable bowel syndrome symptoms, particularly with diarrhea and abdominal pain.

Of particular interest is *Lactobacillus plantarum*, which is reported to produce less gas. Researchers from Sweden examined *L. plantarum* supplementa-

Side Effects: Toxicity is usually only seen in daily doses over 25,000 IU. Side effects include abdominal pain, bone loss, dry skin, fatigue, gingivitis, inflammation of the lips/tongue, hair loss, headaches, high cholesterol, itching, joint pain, liver injury, loss of appetite, nausea, night sweats, and vomiting.

Precautions During Pregnancy: Dosages under 5,000 IU daily are considered safe during pregnancy; the safety of higher dosages is unknown. If you are or intend to become pregnant, do not take more than 8,000 IU of vitamin A daily, as high doses may increase birth defect risk. Vitamin A is normally present in breast milk.

Drug Interactions: Interactions have been reported between vitamin A and atorvastatin, colestipol, corticosteroids, cyclophosphamide, fluvastatin, isotretinoin, lovastatin, medroxyprogesterone, methyltestosterone, mineral oil, minocycline, neomycin, pravastatin, simvastatin, thioridazine, and tretinoin. Interactions have also been described with cancer chemotherapy drugs, oral contraceptives, bile acid binding agents, and cholesterol-lowering drugs. If you are using any of these medications, talk to your doctor prior to taking vitamin A.

tion in sixty patients with IBS in a randomized, placebo-controlled trial. Subjects were given a rose-hip drink that contained *L. plantarum* for four weeks. The authors found that gas was "rapidly and significantly reduced" in the treatment group. They also reported decreased abdominal pain. The subjects were evaluated one year after the study and were found to have maintained better overall gastrointestinal function. The study concluded that *L. plantarum* decreased pain and flatulence in patients with IBS.

Another reason why people with IBS should consider a trial of probiotic therapy is that diarrhea (a common symptom in IBS) can flush healthy bacteria from the bowel, creating an opportunity for potentially harmful bacteria to take hold. Knowing this, some authorities recommend probiotic therapy to restore the normal bacterial balance of the bowel. Early studies have indicated that probiotics may help resolve IBS symptoms by returning the bowel's microflora to a more normal state.

Probiotic formulas vary greatly in levels of the various species of beneficial bacteria. Consult your healthcare provider for the appropriate dosage.

Special Considerations: People with high cholesterol, heart disease, or kidney disease, as well as those at risk for osteoporosis, should speak to their doctor before taking vitamin A. Don't take vitamin A if you have a malabsorption syndrome.

VITAMIN C (ASCORBATE, ASCORBIC ACID)

Vitamin C is one of the body's chief antioxidants. It protects the heart by preventing oxidation of LDL cholesterol, the so-called bad cholesterol implicated in arteriosclerosis. Without vitamin C, your entire body would fall apart, as vitamin C is critical for collagen, the stuff that holds our tissues together. Ascorbic acid also acts as an antihistamine and plays a role in wound healing. So critical is vitamin C that deficiency is linked to cancer, diabetes, heart disease, and asthma. People with IBS have inadequate intakes of many nutrients, including ascorbic acid.

Dietary Sources: Found in many fruits and vegetables and especially abundant in broccoli, Brussels sprouts, citrus fruits, currants, kiwifruit, parsley, red peppers, rose hips, and strawberries.

Dose: Most people take 500 to 1,000 milligrams of vitamin C a day, divided into two to three doses.

Side Effects: While many people can tolerate 2,000 to 4,000 milligrams of vitamin C a day, doses above 2,000 milligrams a day are not recommended and can cause nausea, stomach pain, diarrhea, kidney stones, and copper deficiency. Other side effects include dizziness, excessive urination, flushing, headache, heartburn, insomnia, and vomiting.

Precautions During Pregnancy: If you are pregnant or lactating, speak to your healthcare provider before taking vitamin C.

Drug Interactions: Interactions have been reported between vitamin C and acetaminophen (Tylenol), allopurinol, ampicillin, antibiotics, aspirin, cancer chemotherapy agents, carbidopa, cardec, clozapine, corticosteroids, cyclophosphamide, doxorubicin, epinephrine, indomethacin, isosorbide mononitrate, levodopa, minocycline, nitroglycerine, nitroglyn, oral contraceptives, perhenazine, salsalate, tacrine, tetracycline, thioridazine, and warfarin. If you are using any of these medications, talk to your doctor before taking vitamin C.

Special Considerations: If you have a history of diabetes, kidney stones, kidney failure, glucose-6-phosphate dehydrogenase deficiency, gout, sulfite or tartrazine sensitivity, or have an iron overload problem (hemochromatosis or hemosiderosis), talk to your doctor before taking vitamin C. People who are using blood-thinning medications should also speak to their doctor before taking vitamin C. Since vitamin C supplements can interfere with copper metabolism, it's important to take a copper-containing multivitamin/mineral supplement or copper supplement.

ZINC

Zinc is important for wound healing and plays a critical role in fertility and protein synthesis. Zinc also boosts immune function and acts as an antioxidant. Zinc lozenges may shorten the duration of common cold symptoms. It is used in the treatment of infertility, Wilson's disease, and night blindness. Zinc supplements are important in IBS-associated diarrhea, which can lead to malabsorption-induced zinc deficiency. Other research points to low zinc as a possible cause of fructose malabsorption. In some people, sugar intolerances may be partially or totally responsible for IBS symptoms.

Dietary Sources: Black-eyed peas, eggs, fish, meat, oysters, tofu, and wheat germ.

Dose: Most people who supplement their diet with zinc use 15 milligrams a day, taken with food. Since zinc interferes with copper absorption, most people take extra copper with zinc. Check if your zinc supplement already contains copper before purchasing a separate copper supplement. A daily multivitamin/mineral supplement is also recommended, because zinc competes with other minerals, such as calcium, iron, and magnesium, for absorption.

Side Effects: Side effects are rare and are usually reported with lozenges, which can cause mouth pain, nausea, stomach pain, and vomiting. Zinc dosages over 300 milligrams a day may actually suppress immune function.

Precautions During Pregnancy: If you are pregnant or lactating, talk to your physician before taking zinc.

Drug Interactions: Interactions have been reported between zinc and angiotensin-converting enzyme inhibitors (ACE inhibitors), aspirin, AZT, benazepril, benzamycin, bile acid sequestrants, cancer chemotherapy agents, captopril, chlorhexidine, ciprofloxacin, clindamycin (topical only), corticosteroids (both oral and topical), doxycycline, enoxacin, estrogen, lisinopril, medroxyprogesterone, methyltestosterone, metronidazole (vaginal), minocycline, norfloxacin, ofloxacin, oral contraceptives, penicillamine, quinapril, ramipril, sodium fluoride, tetracycline, thiazide diuretics, valproic acid, and warfarin. If you are using any of these medications, talk to your doctor before taking zinc.

MULTIVITAMIN/MINERAL SUPPLEMENTS

Vitamin and mineral supplements are potentially confusing. Choosing the right supplement is often a matter of trial and error. While there is no substitute for a healthy diet, because vitamins and minerals work best when taken together, a multivitamin/mineral supplement goes a long way toward protecting your health. No matter how healthy or ill you are, I strongly recommend taking a multivitamin/mineral supplement. There are many excellent supplements on the market, but take one that meets (and preferably exceeds) the minimum USDA recommended dietary allowances (RDAs) for vitamins and minerals. With a multivitamin/mineral supplement, you can cover all your bases, achieving the greatest benefit with minimal effort.

This is especially true for people with diarrhea-predominant IBS in order to help prevent the electrolyte losses associated with diarrhea. The most common electrolytes lost in diarrhea are sodium and potassium, which should only be supplemented under the supervision of a physician.

Diarrhea can also lead to malabsorption-induced deficiencies, especially vitamin A and zinc. There is even evidence that a daily multivitamin can reduce anxiety and stress. Even if you don't have a nutritional deficiency, you should consider taking a multivitamin, as there is evidence that people with IBS have inadequate intakes of many nutrients including vitamin A, ascorbic acid, and folic acid.

A WORD OF CAUTION

I want to remind you that many of the drugs we use to treat illness literally have their roots in the plant kingdom. Herbs (or botanicals) contain molecules that, when purified, we call a drug. So, it is important to treat herbs with the same respect—and caution—as our most powerful pharmaceuticals. Through millions of years of trial and error, civilization has found that certain plants have medicinal properties. Only through the emergence of modern chemistry have we been able to isolate and synthesize the natural magic our ancestors discovered. But what do we really mean when we say something is "natural" versus "synthetic"? From a purist perspective, we could say that the only "natural" products are those that are used as they are found in nature. With respect to botanicals, this means ingesting or applying the raw plant product without alteration. We may place this botanical in a pill or drink it as a tea, but the herb remains fundamentally unchanged.

Contrast this with the word "synthetic," which in conventional usage means any material not found in nature. These definitions approximate the meaning of these complex and occasionally controversial words. Most people would agree that plastics are "synthetic" since they do not occur in nature and only result from the manipulations of science. With respect to medicinal herbs, however, the line between natural and synthetic is less clear.

For example, ephedrine can be obtained naturally from the plant *Ephedra sinica* or in synthesized form. Both products contain an identical chemical we call "ephedrine," with the only difference being that one is made in a laboratory and the other is found in a plant. Fundamentally, whether or not your ephedrine comes from a plant or a lab, they both contain the identical active agent, ephedrine. The ephedrine you get from the lab has the same molecular structure as the ephedrine you get from a plant. This is, however, where the similarities end and the differences begin.

The choice between natural and synthetic is often a double-edged sword. A potential problem with some herbal preparations is that, unless the formulation is standardized, the consumer can never be sure how much active ingredient they are taking. This is usually not a problem with isolated or synthesized medications, since strict formulary standards exist. The downside to modern pharmaceuticals is that they often contain additives, like preservatives and colorings, that can spell trouble for someone with IBS. This is a problem you don't usually see with herbs.

Another potential problem with herbal remedies, especially herbal combinations, is that they may contain additional active ingredients that you don't need or could be dangerous. With pharmaceuticals, you know what you're getting: They may contain preservatives and colorings, but you can read about them on the label.

HERBS VERSUS PHARMACEUTICALS

Humans seek predictability, a need that is especially acute for things we ingest. Though we rarely speak about it, it's comforting to know that a glass of cold water will always taste like a glass of cold water and never burn our tongue. We demand the same predictability from the medicines we take and have a strong need to know the risks associated with the pills we swallow. Before we were able to analyze and synthesize medications, we were stuck with what we had. Through experience, we knew what to expect from a particular medicinal herb. However, if that agent had an undesirable side effect, we either didn't take it, accepted the side effect as a part of treatment, or used another botanical.

As technology advanced, we isolated the active ingredients behind these medicinal herbs and were able to synthesize and ultimately manipulate these molecules, often enhancing their therapeutic benefit and eliminating side effects. Molecular biology and organic chemistry also permitted us to develop agents not found in nature, agents that were often more potent than their herbal ancestors. Through standardized testing mandated by agencies like the U.S. Food and Drug Administration, we know what to expect from the majority of pharmaceuticals. In other words, technology and the scientific method allow us to dramatically increase the predictability of the agents we use to treat illness. While it is true that we cannot predict with absolute certainty how a particular individual will react to a given pharmaceutical, through the process of standardized trials we have a good idea of what to expect.

The downside to synthesized pharmaceuticals is that they can result in toxic waste products that are harmful to the environment. From an economic perspective, the manufacturing of new drugs permits pharmaceutical companies to patent and charge exorbitant fees for their products. On the flipside, synthesis has dramatically reduced the economic and environmental costs of some drugs. Nevertheless, there are and probably always will be problems with the way we make and market pharmaceuticals.

I will not deny that much of the resistance of conventional medicine to integrative therapies stems from arrogance and a desire to discourage competition. There are, however, two sides to every story, and while the pharmaceutical industry is far from perfect, if it were not for modern drugs, many people would not be alive today.

The same can be said of the herbal industry—minerals, herbs, and vitamins are big business. Integrative therapies and their associated products represent a multibillion dollar industry. Like the pharmaceutical companies, the herbal industry has its strengths and weaknesses. Medicinal herbs frequently offer consumers products that are not available elsewhere, products that are usually preservative- and additive-free, an important consideration for those with IBS. One of the greatest challenges faced by the herbal industry is standardization. Overall, the herbal industry lacks standardized formulations, and, as mentioned earlier, consumers cannot always be sure how much active ingredient they are ingesting. As for efficacy, we are beginning to see rigorous studies on herbal products published in respected medical journals. While these studies are encouraging, documenting efficacy will take years of research and controversy. Finally, while pharmaceuticals can have a devastating impact on the environment, so too can herbs. For instance, the herb goldenseal *(Hydrastis canadensis)* is endangered because it is overharvested for its medicinal properties. While the herbal industry is far from perfect, think about all the lives herbs have saved through the millennia.

This is the balanced approach to integrative and conventional medicine that I would like to share with you. Keep in mind that the herb that works for one person may not work for you and that some people are even allergic to botanicals. Nevertheless, despite their potential shortcomings, herbs can help people with IBS. Like vitamins and minerals, combined herbal formulations tend to work better than single herbs, a phenomenon herbalists call "orchestration" or "creating a symphony." If you decide to take herbs, I suggest you do so under the guidance of a healthcare professional familiar with herbal therapy. Remember, the line between herb and drug is at best blurred, and many powerful drugs had a humble beginning as a "weed" in somebody's backyard.

Chapter 7

Alternative Therapies for IBS

BS represents a complex interplay between the mind and the body, with anxiety and stress playing leading roles. I am certain almost everyone reading this book knows this is true from personal experience. Throughout this book, I have asked you to do many difficult tasks and ask some hard questions about yourself and your symptoms. I am now asking you the hardest thing of all: I want you to change how you react to IBS. Every time you start to feel symptoms, instead of thinking, "Oh no, I'm going to have an attack," you think, "It's time for me to relax." Not an easy task!

Making the transformation from anxiety to calm is not easy and can take months or years. How you make this transformation is a matter of choice, as there are many paths to choose from. Known as complementary therapies, these paths encompass a wide range of nonpharmacologic treatment options, from acupuncture to hypnosis. While exercising, eating right, and other lifestyle changes are critical to good health, it's equally important to think about how emotions impact your life. You can ponder these thoughts while walking the beach, rock climbing, or with the aid of a therapist—it's up to you. It's probably going to take some trial and error to find which techniques work best for you, but that's half the fun.

It doesn't matter how you relax, whether it's meditating in a Buddhist temple or skydiving—whatever works for you. Which technique you choose is not as important as making a choice, since choosing forces you to pay attention to the mind as well as the body. This book is intended not only to help your IBS, but also to heal old wounds and rid your mind of negative emotional baggage. Each of us deserves to live a good life and be happy with who we are. This is easier said than done, and the road to hap-

Never Underestimate the Power of Suggestion: The Placebo Effect

Before we look at individual therapies, let's examine an area of potential confusion, a problem frequently encountered in research studies on complementary therapies—the "placebo effect." The placebo effect occurs when study subjects receive a placebo (an inert treatment or substance) and nonetheless report improvement because they *believe* the treatment is helping them. One of the major problems in studying a drug or supplement for IBS is that there are high placebo response rates that can range from 30 to 60 percent.

Scientists expect the placebo effect and use statistics to determine when outcome differences between treatment and placebo groups become important or "statistically significant." In other words, what researchers look for is an outcome difference between treatment and placebo groups demonstrating that the treatment provides a measurable benefit beyond what would be expected from the placebo effect alone. By demonstrating this "statistically significant" difference, scientists can assert that the treatment actually works. Sometimes the outcome difference between placebo and treatment groups is so small as to be statistically insignificant; that is, the treatment offers no benefit beyond what would be expected from the placebo effect.

From personal experience, I have learned to respect the power of suggestion. I have successfully used the power of positive thinking with many of my

piness is subject to unforeseen barriers. View this chapter as a road map for making your way around these barriers to enjoy the peace you so rightfully deserve.

WHAT IS INTEGRATIVE MEDICINE?

Integrative medicine can perhaps best be defined as a way of preventing and treating disease using nonconventional techniques. Also known as alternative or complementary medicine, an increasing number of Americans are now embracing these practices and "integrating" them with conventional Western therapies. In the United States, it is estimated that approximately 33 percent of the population has tried some form of complementary therapy; in Australia, this number approaches 50 percent.

It will probably not surprise you to learn that integrative medicine continues to be shunned by many in the mainstream medical community. The patients. Not surprisingly, there is a substantial body of literature affirming that the placebo effect is a potent part of many therapies and that believing something will work can actually influence the outcome. Perhaps one of the best examples of this mind/body phenomenon relates to the immune system—several studies have documented that suggestion under hypnosis can influence immune function in certain individuals with IBS.

Studies have also shown that a physician's attitude toward a particular therapy can influence the efficacy of that therapy. One study compared a group of patients who were offered a treatment by a physician who presented the information in a "positive manner" versus another group who received the information in a "non-positive manner." After two weeks, there was a significant difference in patient satisfaction between the positive and negative groups, as "64 percent of those receiving a positive consultation got better, compared to 39 percent of those who received a negative consultation." The treatment itself was the same in both groups.

The placebo effect represents the healing power of your mind and may be one of the reasons why the treatments discussed in this chapter can help people with IBS. What does this mean for you? If you discover that studies have not supported the use of your favorite therapy, do not stop using that therapy. The placebo effect may be playing a role in your particular case. Remember, what works for one person may not work for another. The only time you should abandon a therapy is if it may cause more harm than good. Bottom line: If the therapy works for you, use it.

good news is that integrative medicine is increasingly recognized by mainstream physicians as an important aspect of American medicine. This is important not because millions of Americans practice some form of integrative medicine, but because some of these therapies really work. While many of these therapies, such as traditional Chinese medicine, have been around for thousands of years, rigorous scientific research into integrative practices is only starting to emerge from its infancy.

This chapter will review several complementary therapies and present the latest scientific research supporting their use. Some of you may be surprised to learn that alternative therapies are nothing new to IBS. In fact, one study found that approximately 16 percent of those with IBS had consulted practitioners of alternative medicine, with 41 percent saying they would consult an alternative medicine practitioner if conventional treatment failed. There is an extensive body of literature supporting the use of alternative therapies for IBS, including acupuncture, hypnosis, and cognitive behavioral therapy. Remember, however, that research on complementary therapies is subject to the same strengths and weaknesses found in all scientific endeavors.

ACUPUNCTURE

Acupuncture has been used in traditional Chinese medicine for over 3,000 years and employs needles strategically placed in "points" on the body. These needles balance the yin (passive) and yang (active) forces and attempt to restore health by increasing energy (known as *qi)* flow through the body's meridians or channels. Sometimes a small electric current is passed through the acupuncture needle to enhance this effect. There are about 365 specific acupuncture points, with several thousand additional points located body wide, particularly on the hands, head, and ears. While acupuncture is used in China to treat virtually any illness, in the West it is primarily employed in treating chronic pain and substance abuse.

Acupuncture has been used successfully to treat diarrhea. Several studies have also shown acupuncture to help depression. In animals, experiments have shown that electroacupuncture (EA) can modulate the neurotransmitter norepinephrine in the brain. Two studies from China, the first in twenty-nine depressed individuals and the other in 241 patients with depression, examined EA stimulation versus amitriptyline, a popular tricyclic antidepressant. The results from both studies showed that the efficacy of acupuncture was equal to that of the antidepressant drug for depression. Electroacupuncture had a better therapeutic effect for anxiety and cognitive disturbances in depressed patients than amitriptyline, and the side effects of EA were much less.

There are, however, questions about the impact of the placebo effect, as one trial on acupuncture and depression found similar results between real and sham acupuncture. In depression, it is suspected that acupuncture influences the manufacture of mood-controlling neurotransmitters, such as serotonin and norepinephrine. Some have found that EA is at least as effective, and with a higher therapeutic index, as amitriptyline. Some success has also been demonstrated in using acupuncture for anxiety.

More research is needed regarding acupuncture and IBS, but these studies are encouraging. People with IBS should consider a trial of acupuncture, and if you have successfully used acupuncture in the past, continue your treatments.

BIOFEEDBACK

Biofeedback trains people to influence bodily functions not normally under conscious control, such as breathing and blood pressure. Biofeedback uses machines to translate these biological functions into signals that the participant can recognize. For instance, in people who have had a stroke, a machine can recognize a muscle twitch in the affected limb and send a signal (such as a "beep") every time the muscle is twitched. By exerting conscious control over the moving the limb with "feedback" from the beeps, the stroke victim may learn to use that limb again.

Biofeedback appears to be especially useful in medical conditions in which psychological factors play a significant role, such as chronic pain, anxiety, insomnia, and asthma. Biofeedback can help asthmatics with relaxation and breath control by training participants to take slow, deep diaphragmatic breaths to reduce anxiety. Biofeedback has been used successfully for people with anismus (anal sphincter spasm) and pelvic muscle dysfunction. In fact, pelvic floor dysfunction biofeedback is 70 to 80 percent effective in some cases. In one study, ten sessions of progressive muscle relaxation training were undertaken by eight people with IBS for a period of eight weeks. Based on daily diaries of gastrointestinal (GI) symptoms collected for four weeks before and four weeks after treatment, the relaxation conditioning produced significant reductions in GI symptoms. Fifty percent of the relaxation group were clinically improved at the end of treatment.

While the ultimate role that biofeedback may play in IBS remains a topic of intense investigation, it is fair to say that biofeedback probably causes beneficial physiologic alterations that contribute to improvements in symptoms.

COGNITIVE-BEHAVIORAL THERAPY (CBT)

CBT combines behavioral and cognitive therapy, two powerful forms of psychotherapy. Behavioral therapy attempts to change how people react to situations by discouraging habituated reactions like anger, depression, or anxiety. While behavioral therapy examines our emotional reactions, cognitive therapy concentrates on how we think and how our thoughts influence the way we feel. "Normalization" of the brain's fear circuit (discussed in Chapter 4) is the mechanism suspected to play a role in the success of cognitive-behavioral therapy for IBS. Cognitive-behavior therapy attempts to attenuate hyperreactivity to gastrointestinal and emotional stimuli in IBS. There are also reports that group cognitive-behavioral therapy helps reduce IBS symptoms.

One study examined the use of CBT in twenty-five individuals with IBS who underwent eight two-hour group sessions over a period of three months. After an average follow-up period of 2.25 years, the abdominal complaints of the patients who underwent treatment were found to improve significantly. The authors also reported that the number of successful coping strategies increased in the treatment group, and the positive changes persisted during follow-up. CBT group treatment helped alleviate IBS symptoms, stimulated new coping strategies, and reduced avoidance behavior.

Another study found that CBT produced significant improvements in the distress associated with bowel symptoms, along with a reduction in anxiety and depression. As for depression, one meta-analysis found that, in four major studies of severely depressed outpatients, cognitive-behavior therapy fared as well as antidepressant medication.

Finally, one study compared a combination of relaxation, thermal biofeedback, and cognitive therapy versus placebo. While the authors reported that there were significant reductions in GI symptoms, anxiety, and depression, there were no significant differences between placebo and treatment groups. However, improved symptoms persisted during the six-month follow-up period. Nevertheless, since several studies have demonstrated that CBT therapy can help people with IBS, CBT is a reasonable option that should be explored by people seeking an alternative IBS treatment.

HYPNOTHERAPY

Hypnosis is an altered state of awareness effected by total concentration on the voice of the therapist, which results in measurable physical, neurophysiological, and psychological changes, producing distortions of emotion, sensation, image, and time. Almost anyone can be hypnotized, and hypnosis has been used successfully for several conditions, ranging from asthma to smoking cessation. Hypnosis is for real, inducing a genuine neurophysiological state that can be demonstrated on an electroencephalogram (EEG).

For people with IBS, a common hypnotic technique is symptom removal by direct suggestion, attempting to modify gut function. Multiple studies have found that hypnosis can help people with IBS. Because people with IBS have lower pain thresholds, researchers have successfully used hypnosis to increase thresholds for gas, urge, stool, and pain. Significant changes in rectal sensitivity were found in patients with diarrhea-predominant IBS, with a trend toward normalization of sensitivity in those with constipation-predominant IBS.

Hypnosis has also been used to "desensitize" the bowel in individuals whose IBS is exacerbated by stress. Many people with IBS have bowels that are exquisitely sensitive to stress. For these individuals, hypnotherapy teaches people how to remain calm during a stressful situation. A common technique is guided imagery, in which the subject relearns how to respond to stress without involving his or her bowels.

Several other hypnotic techniques have also been employed in IBS. Prospective desensitization is a method by which hypnosis is used to manage the stress of anticipated events. For example, a person with IBS is expected to give a public lecture later in the week and knows that this event has the potential to exacerbate his IBS. The therapist may use prospective desensitization to help this individual visualize giving the speech while remaining calm and experiencing "abdominal comfort." Since most people don't have immediate twenty-four-hour access to a hypnotherapist, self-desensitization (self-hypnosis) is often used, with the person learning how to employ visualization to deal with stressful day-to-day events. Many practitioners, in addition to bowel-directed therapy, instill general feelings of well-being and self-worth during sessions. One study examined hypnosis in eight individuals with IBS and reported that all but two of the patients remained relatively symptom free during the three months to twelve years of follow-up. The authors also reported that in the case of the two relapses, symptoms were successfully treated using hypnosis.

With respect to hypnotherapy, there is evidence that some people with IBS may respond better than others. Age may also play a role in hypnotherapy response: One study reported that only 25 percent of those over age fifty had a positive response to hypnosis compared with 100 percent of those under age fifty.

Another study of hypnosis and psychotherapy in thirty patients with severe and refractory IBS utilized "general relaxation." The subjects were asked to place their hand on their abdomen and "feel a sense of warmth and relate this to asserting control over gut function." The psychotherapy group experienced a small but significant improvement in abdominal pain, abdominal distension, and general well-being, but not in bowel habits.

The hypnotherapy patients showed a dramatic improvement in all features, the difference between the two groups being highly significant.

While these results are encouraging for hypnotherapy, they should not discourage you from seeking or continuing to participate in psychotherapy. It's important to remember that IBS is a complex syndrome that can result from multiple causes, which require different treatments tailored to the specific individual.

TRADITIONAL CHINESE MEDICINE (TCM)

Traditional Chinese medicine (TCM) has a rich and ancient history dating back more than 3,000 years. Textbooks have been written on this complex form of medicine that has evolved into several distinct branches. TCM takes a sophisticated view of disease, considering the contributions of both physical and psychological factors. TCM also emphasizes a philosophy of patient education and empowerment, not only to diagnose and treat disease but, more important, to help prevent disease. TCM relies on many different treatment modalities to manage disease: herbal medicine, acupuncture, massage therapy, dietary therapy, and exercise.

The fundamental principles of TCM are Qi, Yin, and Yang. *Qi* is defined as the "vital force," the cumulative energy of all our physical, psychological, and spiritual functions. According to TCM, Qi flows through twelve primary meridians that connect major organs. Health is associated with the free flow of Qi. Disease results when the free flow of Qi through the meridians is hampered, causing too much Qi in some organs and not enough Qi in others. TCM is also concerned with the balance between Yin and Yang, opposite forces that must remain balanced to preserve health.

TCM has been employed for centuries to treat bowel disorders and is commonly used today in China to treat IBS. In the United States, there are thousands of TCM practitioners and colleges that provide training in Chinese medicine. More than thirty states offer licensure to practitioners of TCM.

One study looked at Chinese herbal medicine in 116 IBS patients in a double-blind placebo-controlled trial. Patients in the treatment groups (standard and individualized Chinese herbal medicine) had significant improvement in bowel symptoms. According to the authors, TCM herbal therapy worked because the herbs were designed to "regulate and strengthen bowel function." It was also theorized that these herbs had antianxiety and antispasmodic action. The treatment significantly reduced the interference with life caused by IBS. The authors also reported that only the individualized Chinese herbal medicine treatment group maintained improvement, a finding that reinforces the message that, with most medical conditions, the more individualized the treatment, the better the outcome. This mantra of individualized treatment has been a fundamental tenant of TCM for centuries, a principle that is mercifully being increasingly incorporated into Western practice.

The herbs used in this study were *Codonopsis pilosulae, Agastaches seu pogostemi, Ledebouriellae sesloidis, Coicis lachryma-jobi, Bupleurum chinense, Artemesiae capillaries, Atractylodis macrocephalae, Magnoliae officinalis, Citri reticulatae, Zingiberis offinicinalis, Farina, Peoria cocas, Angelicae dahuricae, Plantaginis, Phellodendri, Glycyrrhizae uralensis, Paeoniac lactiflorae, Saussureae seu vladimirae, Coptidis,* and *Schisandrae.*

What is particularly striking is that both constipation-predominant and diarrhea-predominant IBS subjects were enrolled in the study. Hence, unlike many IBS therapies that tend to work better for one particular form of IBS, TCM may have the potential to benefit people with diarrhea, constipation, or alternating diarrhea-constipation. Equally important, unlike previous studies examining TCM and IBS that were plagued by poor study design, this 1998 trial was well designed and possessed the methodological rigor necessary for its results to be taken seriously by Western medical practitioners.

Another trial compared the aforementioned Chinese herbal preparation against an individually tailored herbal formulation for sixteen weeks in 116 subjects with IBS. The authors found that both standard and individualized treatments were significantly more effective than the placebo treatment in improving bowel symptoms, but individually tailored formulations proved no more effective than the standard treatment. The study did find that the individualized herbal group was better able to maintain improvement once the trial ended. This suggests that individualized herbal treatment did not offer any short-term benefit, but, as in the previous study, it probably offers more long-term benefit.

Given the results of these findings, a trial of TCM is highly recommended for anyone who would like an herbal therapy for IBS. Should you attempt a trial of TCM, make sure you visit an experienced and preferably licensed practitioner as well as review all the herbs used for potential herb-drug interactions. This is especially important as TCM herbal formulations contain numerous herbs that can act synergistically, in both positive and negative ways. Given the number of TCM herbs typically used for IBS, the risk of interactions is high.

Chapter 8

Exercise and IBS

Why exercise? Exercise is important not only to improve your irritable bowel, but also to protect you from this nation's number-one killer: heart disease. Regular exercise, especially aerobic exercise, strengthens your heart and lungs, adding healthy active years to your life. Besides lowering your cholesterol and protecting you from heart disease, a healthy diet coupled with regular exercise reduces your risk for cancer, diabetes, hypertension, and a slew of other illnesses. Exercise helps you sleep better, increases energy levels, and boosts your immune system. Exercise will make you look better and improve your sex life. If you have diabetes, hypertension, depression, fibromyalgia, or virtually any other chronic medical problem, exercise can make your condition more manageable. Even more important, exercise will make you feel great about yourself.

THE BENEFITS OF EXERCISE FOR IBS

With respect to IBS, there is evidence that exercise can help. One study found that women with IBS tended to be less physically active than the rest of the population. Also, within the irritable bowel syndrome group, active women were less likely to report a feeling of incomplete evacuation after a bowel movement than inactive women, and they had less severe somatic symptoms, probably due to lower levels of fatigue. The authors concluded that "physical activity may produce select symptom improvement in women with irritable bowel syndrome."

Another study from the Mayo Clinic examined the impact of diet, exercise, and stress management in fifty-two individuals with IBS. There was a significant reduction in pain and other associated IBS symptoms. Specifically, pain decreased significantly, and patients had normal bowel patterns.

Patients also reported that bloating or distension completely disappeared, and they had less nausea and heartburn. Additionally, patients said that IBS symptoms interfered with their lifestyle less, and visits to physicians for IBS decreased after six months.

Finally, exercise can be especially beneficial for constipation, as constipation is related to inactivity. Many healthcare practitioners routinely recommend exercise for their constipated patients. Even though the benefits of exercise for chronic constipation have been difficult to prove in rigorous scientific trials, clinical experience indicates that exercise can help relieve constipation. One study found that walking was an effective preventative treatment for constipation among men. Another reason to exercise is that physical activity reduces the risk of colon cancer by as much as 50 percent.

As soon as you start to exercise and eat right, as soon as you make a commitment to healthy living, something magical happens: You take control of your life. By living healthy, you say to the world, "I am the master of my fate. I have control, and this is my responsibility." We need this attitude both to beat IBS and to be successful in everything we do.

EXERCISE: THE BASICS

There are three basic exercises that everyone, including people with IBS, should do regularly: aerobic exercise, anaerobic exercise, and stretching. Stretching is the "orphan" of exercise, as few people seem to do it, but it is especially important to help prevent injury. While all three exercises are important, aerobic exercise is probably the most vital for people with IBS. Aerobic exercises like walking, swimming, biking, and running help train your heart and lungs to work as a team. It's the aerobic exercise that will add healthy, active years to your life.

Aerobic Exercise

The type of aerobic exercise you choose depends on your level of physical fitness and personality. If you've been a dedicated couch potato, start by walking for thirty minutes daily. You can walk in your neighborhood, the mall, or the woods. Where you walk depends on where you live and how comfortable you are with walking. If you're in good shape and otherwise healthy, you can walk anywhere. If you have several medical conditions and haven't walked by yourself for some time, walk where other people are present, like the mall. After two weeks of daily walking, increase your walk to an hour every day. As the weeks pass, increase the pace of your walk and include some hills for extra exercise. To make sure you're getting a good workout, you should be breathing a little harder and faster than normal, but not running out of breath or having to stop and rest.

Remember to stay well hydrated during exercise. If you're exercising correctly, chances are you've worked up a sweat. The best replacement fluid is good old-fashioned water. Those expensive "sport" drinks can actually promote dehydration by shifting water to your stomach to digest their sweeteners and electrolytes. What can happen is that you become increasingly dehydrated as your stomach tries to dilute the concentrated drink. So, during exercise, take frequent but small sips of water to stay hydrated. Salt and electrolyte replacement is usually only needed by heavily perspiring athletes.

After a couple of months of dedicated walking, try biking, swimming, or joining an aerobics class. Once again, the type of activity you choose depends on your fitness level, personality, and where you live. If you live in a large city, biking may not be a realistic option, and you might consider joining a gym, where you can swim or take an aerobics class. Aerobics classes come in all shapes and sizes, so you should have no problem finding a class that's right for you. Since swimming, biking, and aerobics tend to be more intense than walking, you won't have to do them as often to stay in shape; thirty to forty-five minutes every other day should be adequate.

As with any type of exercise, your mantra should be "go slow and work your way up." For moderate-level aerobic exercise, you want to be breathing a little faster than you would while walking. Don't be embarrassed to rest if you need to, as it's better to gradually develop aerobic strength rather than overwork and potentially injure your body. There are formulas for calculating target aerobic heart rate, which for most people are unnecessary. When exercising, pay attention to what your body tells you. You know you're getting a good workout if you're breathing fast but can still carry on a conversation. If you can't catch your breath or complete a sentence, you're exercising too hard and need to slow down. Unless you're in excellent, competitive-level shape, leave the heart-pounding, body-bashing stuff to the athletes. For people with IBS who want to stay fit and do not intend to engage in high-intensity sports, I recommend sticking to moderate-level aerobic exercise, which offers similar health benefits to high-intensity exercise without the risk of injury.

Anaerobic Exercise

For most people, anaerobic exercise means weight lifting. Like aerobic exercise, weight lifting comes in all shapes and sizes. Pumping iron will give you the strength necessary for aerobic exercise. Another important health benefit of weight lifting is that you preserve muscle mass; this becomes increasingly critical as we age, since our bodies normally replace muscle with fat. By lifting, you prevent this natural decline in muscle mass and protect yourself against conditions like diabetes—muscle consumes more sugar than fat, and this is why muscular people have less risk of diabetes than those who are obese.

The main reason to pump iron, however, is that the more muscle you have, the more you'll be able to run, walk, bike, or whatever activity you choose. The good news is you don't have to look like a bodybuilder or bench press 300 pounds to benefit from weight training. How much weight you lift depends on your fitness level and what you're trying to accomplish. I recommend starting with light weights and working your way up to moderate weights, leaving the heavy stuff for the bodybuilders.

"Light weights" means different things to different people, and what is light for an eighteen year old is probably dangerous for an eighty year old. How much weight you start with is going to involve some trial and error. Ideally, you should feel resistance when lifting, with the weight neither too easy nor too hard to lift. You should not feel pain—if you feel pain, stop lifting immediately, rest a minute, and then resume lifting with a lighter weight.

If you're a true beginner, I recommend starting with five to twenty pounds for arm/chest/shoulder exercises and twenty to seventy pounds for leg exercises. There are many excellent books on weight lifting available in bookstores that can show you the basic exercises. While quality exercise equipment for home use is available, it can be expensive. Since all the machinery needed to perform multiple exercises can be found in most gyms, the gym is probably the best choice for beginners. There's also a safety issue: If you injure yourself, it helps to have other people around rather than being home alone.

I strongly recommend that if you're new to weight lifting, you join a gym and enlist the services of a personal trainer. This may seem expensive at first; however, a personal trainer knows which exercises and weight loads are right for you and will teach you how to lift correctly and safely.

IBS and the Athlete

If you like to ski, climb, mountain bike, or engage in any other strenuous activity, working your body hard is not a bad idea, as long as you're an otherwise healthy, well-conditioned individual. In other words, IBS is no excuse for athletic mediocrity. Before you join the local rugby team, make sure you've been performing mid- to high-level aerobic exercise, along with some weight training and stretching thrown in for good measure. Don't just roll out of bed one morning and decide that, after ten years of sitting in front of the TV, you're going to run marathons. This is not only a good way to get hurt, but you actually risk your life.

If you've been exercising regularly and you have no other medical problems that would stop you from exercising, then there's no reason why you can't push yourself to the next level. Of course, it's always a good idea to talk to your doctor before embarking on an exercise program, especially one where you intend to push your body hard. Which exercises you choose depend on your personality and availability. With aerobic exercise, try to mix things up and not do the same exercise every day. If you perform the same exercise daily, your body adapts and you don't get an effective workout. So, run on the track or treadmill one day, pound the stair-climbing machine at the gym the next day, rest one day, then bike the next day—cross-training is good for your body.

If you're serious about exercise, I strongly recommend joining a gym, where you will find all the equipment you need and trained professionals to show you how to use it safely and properly. As usual, always check with your doctor before starting an anaerobic or aerobic exercise program.

Once you've learned how to lift properly, you can go it alone. At the gym, you can also interact with like-minded individuals, supporting one another and learning from one another's successes and mistakes.

Remember, weight lifting is for everyone. Even people with severe medical conditions and disabilities can benefit from a properly tailored weight-lifting program. Multiple studies have found that regular aerobic and anaerobic exercise adds healthy years to one's life and can help prevent and ameliorate medical problems like diabetes and high blood pressure. Exercise is especially beneficial for individuals with chronic pain problems like rheumatoid arthritis or fibromyalgia, and multiple studies have demonstrated that people experience less pain when they exercise regularly.

The Orphan: Stretching

Stretching is the orphan of exercise—everybody talks about it, but few do it. Stretching is nonetheless critical and probably the most important part of your exercise regimen. The older we get, the more brittle we become and the more likely we are to be injured, especially during exercise. Stretching keeps your ligaments, tendons, and muscles strong and flexible. The stronger your muscles, the better your performance, whether you're playing football or casting a fly into your favorite stream. The same goes for flexibility—the more flexible you are, the better your performance and the less risk of injury. Some say stretching is best done before exercising, while others say afterward is better. The available books on exercise will only add to your confusion about how, when, and why to stretch. Many people find stretching boring and don't do it at all. Fortunately, there are ways to make stretching more interesting. For instance, yoga is one of the best all-around exercises you can do, and I say this from personal experience. Yoga combines strength, flexibility, and balance—all essential to athletic performance. When I started doing yoga, my skiing skills zoomed up several notches. For those of you who think yoga is not really exercise, try sitting "Indian style" with one hand between your legs pressed firmly to the floor and lift yourself off the ground. No easy feat! Yoga comes in many different forms to suit every need—whether you're an Olympic athlete or a paraplegic, yoga has something to offer you.

Perhaps most important, yoga will teach you how to breathe. "Teach me how to breathe?" you may be asking, "Hey! I've been breathing all my life." However, there is good breathing and bad breathing. What every person with IBS must do in this high-stress world is learn to relax, a tall order for many. This is where yoga enters the picture. With yoga, not only will you be perfecting your balance, flexibility, and strength, you'll also be helping your lungs by relieving stress and soothing your soul. I recommend fifteen to thirty minutes of yoga before exercise.

If you're stressed out, try some peace and quiet with yoga or tai chi. Some of you may want more intensity: Karate, judo, and kickboxing emphasize the same essentials as yoga, but with a different perspective. If you want to "sweat out" your stress or build up your confidence in handling stressful situations, then one of these martial arts may be what you're looking for. Excellent books and videos can show you the moves, or you can hire a private instructor or take a group class. How you learn depends on how much you're willing to spend and on your unique personality. My advice is to just do it!

EXERCISE FOR LIFE

Why exercise? I believe it's vital to revisit this question. On the most basic level, exercise will keep you healthy, help you live a long life, and improve your IBS. Regular exercise can help you stay slim and avoid obesity—obesity dramatically increases your risk for diabetes, heart disease, hypertension, arthritis, and many other illnesses. Equally important, exercise will allow you to do the things you want to do in life. Exercise will make you feel good about yourself, something many people, with or without IBS, have a problem with. Even more critical, exercise can help you take control of your life and health.

Chapter 9

Pharmacological Management

Despite our best efforts, there will always be some people with irritable bowel syndrome who will need medication to control their symptoms. Drugs are certainly not the best way to treat any medical condition; however, for some people, medications will remain an occasional, or permanent, fact of life. There is no doubt that medications can cause problems of their own. What I personally find disturbing, however, is when authors slander IBS medications, calling them poisons and accusing them of doing more harm than good. While it is true that many medications have potentially disturbing side effects, that some physicians rely too heavily on medications to treat IBS, and that many patients are over-medicated, it is also true that there are millions of people who have been helped by IBS pharmacotherapy.

Knowledge is power, and the more you know about the drugs you take, the more effective they will be for you. While the purpose of this book is to help you become medication-free or dramatically reduce the amount of medication you are taking, this chapter can help you avoid drug-related side effects while extracting the most benefit from pharmaceuticals.

In many ways, conventional and complementary therapies for IBS are not very different. Both rely on a positive and trusting relationship between the patient and healthcare professional. In fact, studies have shown that a positive physician-patient relationship favorably impacts IBS treatment and results in fewer hospitalizations. As in alternative medicine, diet plays a major role in the conventional treatment of IBS, along with stress management and psychotherapy, when indicated. Where traditional and alternative therapies diverge is in the use of medications. Support, reassurance, and dietary modification are, for the vast majority of patients, first-line treatment modalities. When these interventions fail or do not produce a satisfactory response, many doctors will turn to pharmacologic therapy.

In medicine, there is usually a substantial body of evidence supporting the use of pharmaceuticals for a particular condition, such as asthma, diabetes, or heart disease. IBS, however, was for years the exception—many of the drugs previously used lacked an adequate number of quality studies to definitively support their use. This is beginning to change, and we now have extensive trials examining many of these agents. These studies have demonstrated that many of these agents are safe and effective in the treatment of IBS.

Like the syndrome itself, the field of IBS pharmacologic management is complex. To simplify our discussions, IBS agents can be divided into anticholinergics, antispasmodics, antidepressants and opiods, and prokinetics. Laxatives are also commonly given for IBS-related constipation. We will examine each of these individually, drawing out their strengths and weaknesses.

ANTICHOLINERGICS

Anticholinergics work by blocking the neurotransmitter acetylcholine, which triggers smooth muscle contraction and is often prescribed for people with diarrhea-predominant IBS and/or abdominal pain. Anticholinergics are also used to abort acute abdominal pain or to prevent symptoms prior to a meal. In people with IBS, anticholinergics are essentially antispasmodics; however, it is because of their unique mechanism of action that they are discussed separately. While anticholinergics effectively relieve symptoms, their use is limited by a high side effect profile.

AGENTS: Dicyclomine (Antispas, Bemote, Bentyl, Bentylol, Byclomine, Dibent, Dilomine, Di-Spaz, Formulex, Neoquess, Or-Tyl), **hyoscyamine** (Anaspaz, Cystospaz, Cystospaz-M, Donnamar, ED-SPAZ, Gastrosed, Levbid, Levsin, Levsin Drops, Levsin/SL, Levsinex Timecaps, Neoquess), and **atropine** (Atropair, Atropen, Atropisol, Isopto Atropine, I-Tropine, Sal-Tropine).

Side Effects: Anticholinergics are plagued by side effects that include anxiety, blurred vision, confusion, constipation, dizziness, drowsiness, dry mouth, fast heart rates, hallucinations, impotence, insomnia, rash, urinary retention, and vomiting.

Absolute Contraindications: Do not use anticholinergics if you have abnormal heart rhythms, asthma, heart disease, narrow angle glaucoma, gastrointestinal atony/obstruction, myasthenia gravis, paralytic ileus, prostate enlargement, thyrotoxicosis, toxic megacolon, or ulcerative colitis.

Drug Interactions: Amantadine, ketoconazole, H1-antihistamines, levodopa, MAOIs, neuroleptics, phenothiazines, rimantadine, tacrine, and tricyclic antidepressants.

ANTISPASMODICS AND NARCOTICS

Antispasmodics help prevent bowel spasms by decreasing gastrointestinal peristalsis and are most commonly used for abdominal pain/cramping, bloating, and diarrhea. If someone is considered refractory to traditional antispasmodic therapy, then a trial of nitrates may be used. Nitrates act by directly relaxing smooth muscle. Loperamide (Imodium) and diphenoxylate (Lomotil, Lonox, and Motofen) are the quintessential antispasmodics often used to treat diarrhea. These agents are reported to reduce the number of bowel movements and improve the consistency of stool.

One meta-analysis reviewed twenty-six randomized, double-blind, placebo-controlled trials and found that antispasmodics helped alleviate pain and improved overall feelings of wellness. Trials involving cimetropium bromide, octilium bromide, pinaverium bromide, dicyclomide bromide, mebeverine, trimebutine, peppermint oil, and hyoscine were included. According to the authors, all myorelaxants (muscle relaxants) were significantly better than placebo with respect to pain control and global assessment. This same trial, however, failed to find any significant improvement in bloating and constipation. Adverse reactions occurred in 6 percent of the treatment groups, with the most common side effects being found in peppermint oil (heartburn) and dicyclomide bromide (blurred vision, dizziness, and dry mouth). Five drugs proved to be particularly effective in patients with IBS: cimetropium bromide, pinaverium bromide, trimebutine, octilium bromide, and mebeverine. For pain improvement, the top three drugs were cimetropium bromide, octilium bromide, and pinaverium bromide.

In 2001, antispasmodics were evaluated in another meta-analysis that reviewed the effectiveness of cimetropium bromide, hyoscine butyl bromide, mebeverine, otilium bromide, pinaverium bromide, and trimebutine. The authors found that 56 percent of patients in the treatment groups reported increased global improvement scores and 53 percent reported improved symptoms. Abdominal distension/bloating improved in 44 percent of the treatment groups, but no significant improvements were observed for diarrhea or constipation. According to this study, the top three smooth muscle relaxants with respect to global improvement were trimebutine, cimetropium, and otilium. From the data, it also appears that cimetropium, pinaverium, and otilium had the most impact on abdominal pain.

In the final analysis, these studies support the use of smooth muscle relaxants for treating IBS-related abdominal pain and perhaps bloating.

Narcotics inhibit the action of intestinal smooth muscle, thereby reducing bowel motility. Narcotics are the drugs of last resort for the treatment of IBS because of their high side effect profile and risk of abuse and dependency. There are, however, opiates such as loperamide and diphenoxylate that are not absorbed by the bowel and have been used successfully to treat diarrhea. Additionally, one study showed that loperamide may benefit people who have rectal urgency.

AGENT: Loperamide (Imodium, Imodium A-D, Kaopectate II, Maalox Anti-Diarrheal, Pepto Diarrheal Control).

Side Effects: Abdominal pain, constipation, dizziness, dry mouth, fatigue, fever, nausea, toxic megacolon, rash, and vomiting.

Absolute Contraindications: Do not use loperamide if you have diarrhea caused by an infection, are constipated, or have a history of pseudomembranous colitis.

AGENT: Diphenoxylate (Logen, Lomanate, Lomotil, Lonox).
Side Effects: Abdominal distension/pain, dizziness, dry mouth, fatigue, nausea, rash, and vomiting.

Absolute Contraindications: Do not use diphenoxylate if you have diarrhea caused by an infection, a history of pseudomembranous colitis, or obstructive jaundice.

Drug Interactions: Alcohol, barbiturates, MAOIs, and narcotics. If you are using any of these medications, speak to your physician before using diphenoxylate.

ANTIDEPRESSANTS AND BENZODIAZEPINES

One of the most important advances in the treatment of IBS stems from research showing that psychiatric medications can help people with IBS regardless of whether they have a psychiatric disorder. Likewise, for individuals with IBS and psychiatric issues, treatment with these agents is very effective. The two major types of antidepressants used to treat IBS are the older tricyclic antidepressants (TCAs) and the newer selective serotonin reuptake inhibitors (SSRIs). Antianxiety or anxiolytic agents are also commonly used in IBS, including the benzodiazepines.

If your physician places you on an antidepressant, don't immediately assume this is because he or she believes you are depressed or your symptoms are "in your head." Thanks in part to the revolutionary Brain-Gut Model, antidepressants are emerging as a first-line therapy for IBS in people with or without a psychiatric disorder. Enhancing the role of antidepressants is evidence of IBS-related serotonin dysfunction and, because of this, agents that act on the serotonin system, such as the SSRIs, are now commonly employed against IBS.

Many people with IBS also benefit from antidepressants because these agents have anticholinergic and painkilling action. SSRIs are emerging as the preferred antidepressant for IBS given their low side effect profile and safety. It is suspected that these agents work by "normalizing" the brain's fear circuit. As discussed in Chapter 4, central nervous system (CNS) and enteric nervous system (ENS) dysfunction are implicated as playing a leading role in causing IBS. It is theorized that antidepressants and benzodiazepines normalize these interactions, thereby relieving IBS symptoms. A major mediator of this brain-gut dysfunction is corticotropin-releasing factor (CRF); antidepressants and benzodiazepines inhibit CRF action. The benefits of these agents are multiplied in those individuals who also suffer from depression and panic disorder. Studies also demonstrate that antidepressants can influence bowel transit time and improve bowel function while providing an enhanced sense of well-being.

While TCAs help reduce IBS symptoms, pain thresholds appear to remain unchanged. There are, however, several small studies that demonstrate that low-dose tricyclics help abdominal pain. One study from Australia examined amitriptyline in forty people with IBS: It was found to be significantly more effective than placebo in producing global improvement, increasing feelings of well-being, reducing abdominal pain, and increasing satisfaction with bowel movements. A recently published meta-analysis found that TCAs are effective in treating some people with IBS, especially with respect to global improvement.

Despite promising theoretical value, experience with SSRIs is mixed. Several reports indicate that SSRIs are effective in IBS; however, in some people, SSRIs may exacerbate symptoms. Benzodiazepines are useful in people with anxiety and IBS but are weak depression fighters. If anxiety and depression coexist, a combined approach with benzodiazepines and antidepressants is often used. Both TCAs and SSRIs have emerged as standard therapy for depression and IBS. The one class of agents I would avoid, however, is the monoamine oxidase inhibitors (MAOIs), such as isocarboxazid (Marplan), phenelzine (Nardil), and tranylcypromine (Parnate). While MAOIs are effective antidepressants, they have multiple drug interactions that limit their use.

A new drug for IBS is tegaserod, a partial serotonin agonist. One study reported that tegaserod reduced sensitivity to rectal distension. Tegaserod has also been reported to shorten transit time in the colon and small intestine, increase the frequency of bowel movements, and soften stools. One study evaluated tegaserod in 881 people with IBS and found that tegaserod offered rapid and sustained relief of abdominal pain and constipation and is also well tolerated. Other emerging agents include kappa-opioid agonists and neurokinin antagonists.

BENZODIAZEPINES: Alprazolam (Xanax), **diazepam** (Diastat, Valium), and **lorazepam** (Ativan).

Side Effects: Anxiety, blurred vision, confusion, constipation, depression, diarrhea, dizziness, dry mouth, fatigue, hallucinations, headache, heart rhythm abnormalities, hypertension, insomnia, liver problems, loss of appetite, low blood pressure, nausea, respiratory depression, ringing in ears, rash, tremors, and vomiting.

Contraindications: Do not use benzodiazepines if you have a history of psychosis, acute narrow-angle glaucoma, or are currently using itraconazole, ketoconazole, or nefazadone.

Drug Interactions: Carbamazepine, cimetidine, ciprofloxacin, clarithromycin, clozapine, delavirdine, digoxin, disulfiram, erythromycin, ethanol, fluconazole, fluoxetine, fluvoxamine, grapefruit juice, isoniazid, itraconazole, ketoconazole, levodopa, metoprolol, nefazadone, omeprazole, phenytoin, quinolones, rifampin, and troleandomycin. If you are taking any of these medications, speak to your doctor before using a benzodiazepine.

Special Considerations: Do not suddenly stop taking a benzodiazepine without your doctor's permission. Sudden discontinuation can cause withdrawal symptoms. Ask your doctor if you need to have your liver function tested. Also ask your doctor if you can drive or perform other potentially hazardous activities while using a benzodiazepine. Avoid alcohol or other sedating medication when taking a benzodiazepine.

SSRIs: Fluoxetine (Prozac), paroxetine (Paxil), and sertraline (Zoloft).

Side Effects: Agitation, anxiety, chest pain, constipation, delusions, diarrhea, dizziness, dry mouth, fatigue, flatulence, hallucinations, headache, hot flashes, insomnia, loss of appetite, low blood sugar, muscle/joint pain, nausea, nervousness, palpitations, rash, seizures, sexual dysfunction, tremor, vision problems, vomiting, and weight loss.

Contraindications: Do not use SSRIs if you are using or have stopped using a MAOI in the last two weeks. Nor should you start to use a MAOI until two weeks after you have stopped using an SSRI.

Drug Interactions: Alprazolam, astemizole, atorvastatin, benzodiazepines, beta blockers, bumetanide, buspirone, carbamazepine, clomipramine, coumadin, cyproheptadine, desipramine, dexfenfluramine, dextromethorphan, diazepam, digoxin, diuretics, doxepin, fenfluramine, fluoxetine, furosemide, haloperidol, imipramine, isocarboxazid, lithium, lovastatin, MAOIs, metroprolol, nortriptylline, phenelzine, phenobarbital, phenothiazines, phenytoin, propranolol, quinidine, selegiline, simvastatin, sotalol, TCAs, terfenadine, theophylline, torsemide, tranylcypromine, trazodone, tryptophan, and warfarin. If you are using any of these medications, speak to your physician before using a SSRI.

Special Considerations: SSRIs may take four to six weeks to be effective.

TRICYCLIC ANTIDEPRESSANTS (TCAs): Amitriptyline (Elavil), **desipramine** (Norpramin, Pertofrane), **doxepin** (Sinequan), **imipramine** (Tofranil), and **nortriptyline** (Aventyl, Pamelor).

Side Effects: Abdominal cramps, abnormal heart rhythms, anxiety, bleeding, blood disorders, blurred vision, confusion, constipation, dry mouth/eyes, headache, hepatitis, increased appetite, insomnia, memory problems, nausea, nightmares, palpitations, panic, rash, sedation, stuffy nose, tremor, vomiting, urinary retention, weakness, and weight gain. Side effects are more common with primary tricyclics; secondary tricyclics may have less side effects.

Contraindications: Do not use TCAs if you are also using MAOIs or recently had a heart attack.

Drug Interactions: Anticholinergics, barbiturates, bethanidine, carbamazepine, chlorpropamide, cimetidine, clonidine, coumadin, debrisoquin, diltiazem, epinephrine, ethanol, fluoxetine, fluvoxamine, guanabenz, guanethidine, guanadrel, guanfacine, indinavir, lithium, moclobemide, MAOIs, neuroleptics, norepinephrine, paraoxetine, phenylephrine, propxoyphene, quinidine, rifampin, ritonavir, sulfonylureas, and warfarin. If you are using any of these medications, talk to your doctor before using a TCA.

Special Considerations: Ask your doctor if you need to have your blood checked for hepatitis or other blood problems. You may also need to have your heart checked with an EKG. TCAs usually take four to six weeks to work and should not be discontinued without your doctor's permission. Do not use alcohol or other depressants while using TCAs. Driving or other potentially hazardous activities must be performed with extreme caution while using TCAs. Some people may feel dizzy after rising too quickly from sitting or lying down: if this happens to you, try to arise slowly. Ask your doctor if you need to wear sunscreen while using TCAs.

PROKINETIC AGENTS

Prokinetic agents enhance gut motility and are usually used for people with constipation-predominant IBS. Commonly used prokinetic agents include metoclopramide, domperidone, and, until recently, cisapride. Studies on metoclopramide have yielded disappointing results, and this drug is not recommended for IBS due to its high side effect profile. Similar disappointing results have been reported for domperidone. Cisapride (Propulsid) used to be a popular and effective prokinetic agent, but was taken off the market in 2000 because of potentially lethal cardiac side effects. One study reported that cisapride reduced abdominal bloating and pain and increased more "normal" stool. But this study also found that people with diarrhea-predominant IBS experienced an exacerbation when using these drugs. With the removal of cisapride from the market, there are presently no prokinetic agents available that have demonstrated efficacy in treating IBS.

LAXATIVES

Laxatives are usually used to treat constipation. There are two basic types of laxatives: stimulatory and osmotic. Stimulatory laxatives cause bowel peristalsis and influence gastrointestinal water and electrolyte secretion. Osmotic laxatives work by introducing a nonabsorbable agent into the colon, which causes fluid to be drawn into the colon and stool, thereby increasing the stool's bulk and making it easier to pass. Two common osmotic laxatives are lactulose and sorbitol, both of which use a nonabsorbable sugar. Other common osmotic laxatives include magnesium citrate, milk of magnesia, and polyethylene glycol. Senna is also sometimes used as a stimulant laxative, but its use is limited by side effects, mostly tachyphylaxis (a rapid development of tolerance to a repeatedly administered drug). These agents should be avoided because they may damage the bowel's nervous system.

OSMOTIC LAXATIVES: Lactulose (Acilac, Cephulac, Cholac, Chronulac, Comalose-R, Constilac, Constulose, Duphalac, Enulose, Evalose, Gen-Lac, Hepatalac, Lactulax, Laxilose) and **sorbitol**.

Side Effects: Abdominal pain, bloating, burping, diarrhea, flatulence, nausea, and vomiting.

Contraindications: Do not use osmotic laxatives if you are on a low-galactose diet.

Special Considerations: Do not use with other laxatives. Ask your doctor if you should have you blood checked while using an osmotic laxative.

STIMULATORY LAXATIVES: Senna (Black Draught, Dr. Caldwell's Senna Laxative, Fletcher's Castoria, Gentlax, Glysennid, Senexon, Seena-Gen, Sennatab, Senokot, Senokotxtra, Senolax, X-Prep).

Side Effects: Abdominal cramps, diarrhea, loss of appetite, low calcium/potassium, nausea, and vomiting.

Contraindications: Do not use stimulatory laxatives if you have a history of bowel obstruction, fecal impaction, active abdominal pain/nausea/ vomiting, or gastrointestinal bleeding.

Drug Interactions: Interactions have been reported with anticoagulants. If you are using a blood thinner, speak to your doctor before taking a stimulatory laxative.

Special Considerations: Even though stimulatory laxatives are available over the counter, they should be avoided by people with IBS and only be used under the guidance of a healthcare professional.

Afterword

I hope this book has helped you learn about irritable bowel syndrome and the various roles that diet, emotions, and supplements/alternative therapies can play in its management. IBS may seem to be simply a gastrointestinal problem; however, after reviewing the most up-to-date scientific literature, it is increasingly clear that, for many people, IBS has a lot more to do with how they live and how they feel. While there are clearly physiological abnormalities observed in IBS, we now know that diet, emotions, and lifestyle can play pivotal roles. For some people, diet may be to blame. For others, emotions may be a leading factor. Some people may learn that they don't even have IBS but rather have another medical condition such as lactose intolerance that is causing their symptoms.

Much of the advice in this book can be used to make your life healthier. Take control of your IBS—don't let your IBS to take control of you! While a proper diet coupled with the judicious use of supplements can help add healthy years to your life, equally important is living healthy. What I mean by "living healthy" is embracing a program of a good diet, adequate sleep, regular exercise, and a balanced, positive outlook toward life. Not only will healthy living help you beat IBS, it will empower you to solve any other health problems you may have, such as diabetes, hypertension, and heart disease. Learn to control your life and embrace a daily program of healthy living and you will not only overcome IBS, but you will also become the master of your own destiny and enjoy the symptom-free life you so richly deserve.

References

Chapter 1

Bearcroft, C.P., Perrett, D., Farthing, M.J.G., "Postprandial plasma 5-hydroxytryptamine in diarrhea predominate irritable bowel syndrome: a pilot study," *Gut*, 42 (1998): 42–46.

Bose, M., Nickols, C., Feakins, R., et al., "5-Hydroxytryptamine and enterochromaffin cells in the irritable bowel syndrome," *Gastroenterology*, 118 (2000): SA2949.

Creed, F., Craig, T., Farmer, R., "Functional abdominal pain, psychiatric illness, and life events," *Gut*, 29 (1988): 235–242.

Feldman, M., Scharschmidt, B.F., Sleisenger, M.H., *Sleisenger & Fordtran's Gastrointestinal and Liver Disease*. 6th Edition. (New York: W.B. Saunders, 1998) 1536.

Harvey, R.F., Mauad, E.C., Brown, A.M., "Prognosis in the irritable bowel syndrome: a 5-year prospective study," *The Lancet*, (1987): 963–65.

Horwitz, B.J., Fisher, R.S., "The Irritable Bowel Syndrome," *New England Journal of Medicine*, 2001; 344: 1846–1850.

Kane, S.V., Sable, K., Hanauer, S.B., "The menstrual cycle and its effects on inflammatory bowel disease and irritable bowel syndrome: a prevalence study," *Am. J. Gastroenterology*, 93 (1998):1867–72.

Chapter 2

Bonaz, B.L., Baciu, M., Papillon, E., et al., "Central processing of rectal pain in IBS patients: an fMRI study," *Gastroenterology*, 97 (2002): 654–661.

Creed, F., Craig, T., Farmer, R., "Functional abdominal pain, psychiatric illness, and life events," *Gut*, 29 (1988): 235–242.

Evans, P.R., Bennett, E.J., Young-Tae, B., et al., "Jejunal sensorimotor dysfunction in irritable bowel syndrome: clinical and psychosocial features," *Gastroenterology,* 110 (1996): 393–404.

Feldman, M., Scharschmidt, B.F., Sleisenger, M.H., *Sleisenger & Fordtran's Gastrointestinal and Liver Disease.* 6th Edition. (New York: W.B. Saunders, 1998) 1538–9.

Feldman, M., Scharschmidt, B.F., Sleisenger, M.H., *Sleisenger & Fordtran's Gastrointestinal and Liver Disease.* 6th Edition. (New York: W.B. Saunders, 1998) 1538.

Hebden, J.M., Blackshaw, E., D'Amato, M., et al., "Abnormalities of GI transit in bloated irritable bowel syndrome: effect of bran on transit and symptoms," *Am. J. Gastroenterology,* 97 (2002): 2315–20.

King, T.S., Elia, M., Hunter, J.O., "Abnormal colonic fermentation in irritable bowel syndrome," *The Lancet,* 352 (1998): 1187–89.

Silverman, D.H.S., Munakata, J.A., Ennes, H., et al., "Regional cerebral activity in normal and pathological perception of visceral pain," *Gastroenterology,* 112 (1997): 64–72.

Sullivan, M., Cohen, S., Snape, W.J., Jr., "Colonic myoelectrical activity in irritable bowel syndrome: effect of eating and anticholinergics," *N. Engl. J. Med.,* 298 (1978): 878–83.

Waxman, D., "The irritable bowel: a pathological or a psychological syndrome?" *J. Royal Soc. Med.* 81 (1988): 718–720.

Whitehead, W.E., Engel, B.T., Schuster, M.M., "Irritable bowel syndrome: physiological and psychological differences between diarrhea-predominant and constipation-predominant patients," *Dig. Dis. Sci.,* 25 (1980): 404–413.

Whitehead, W.E., Palsson, O.S., "Is rectal pain sensitivity a biological marker for irritable bowel syndrome: psychological influences on pain perception," *Gastroenterology,* 115 (1998): 1263–71.

Chapter 3

Gee, M.I., Grace, M.G., Wensel, R.H., et al., "Nutritional status of gastroenterology outpatients: comparison of inflammatory bowel disease with functional disorders," *J. Am. Diet Assoc.,* 85 (1985): 159.

Horwitz, B.J., Fisher, R.S., "The irritable bowel syndrome," *New England Journal of Medicine,* 344 (2001): 1846–1850.

Lydiard, R.B., "Irritable bowel syndrome, anxiety, and depression: what are the links?" *J. Clin. Psychiatry,* 62 suppl. 8 (2001): 38–45.

Chapter 4

Ballenger, J.C., Davidson, J.R.T., Lecrubier, Y., et al., "Consensus statement on depression, anxiety, and functional gastrointestinal disorders," *J. Clin. Psychiatry,* 62 suppl. 8 (2001): 48–51.

Creed, F., Craig, T., Farmer, R., "Functional abdominal pain, psychiatric illness, and life events," *Gut,* 29 (1988): 235–242.

Dancey, C.P., Whitehouse, A., Painter, J., et al., "The relationship between hassles, uplifts, and irritable bowel syndrome: a preliminary study," *J. Psychosomatic Res.,* 39 (1995): 827–832.

"Experimental studies on the irritable colon," *Am. J. Med.,* 10 (1951) 60.

Ford, M.J., Camilleri, M., Zinsmeister, A.R., et al., "Psychosensory modulation of colonic sensation in the human transverse and sigmoid colon," *Gastroenterology,* 109 (1995): 1772–80.

Gomborone, J., Dewsnap, P., Libby, G., et al., "Abnormal illness attributes in patients with irritable bowel syndrome," *J. Psychosom. Res.,* 40 (1996): 95–104.

Guthrie, E., Creed, F., Dawson, D., et al., "A controlled trial of psychological treatment for the irritable bowel syndrome," *Gastroenterology,* 100 (1991): 450–57.

Guthrie, E., Creed, F., Dawson, D., et al., "A randomized controlled trial of psychotherapy in patients with refractory irritable bowel syndrome," *Br. J. Psychiatry,* 163 (1993): 315–321.

Johnson, R., Jacobsen, B.K., Forde, O.H., "Associations between symptoms of irritable colon and psychological and social conditions and lifestyle," *Br. Med. J.,* 292 (1986): 1633–35.

Langeluddecke, P.M., "Psychological aspects of irritable bowel syndrome," *Aust. N. Z. J. Psychiatry,* 19 (1985): 218–226.

Lydiard, R.B., Fossey, M.D., Marsh, W., et al., "Prevalence of psychiatric disorders in patients with irritable bowel syndrome," *Psychosomatics,* 34 (1993): 229–34.

Lydiard, R.B., "Anxiety and the irritable bowel syndrome: psychiatric, medical, or both?" *J. Clinical Psychiatry,* 58 suppl. 3 (1997): 51–58.

Lydiard, R.B., "Irritable bowel syndrome, anxiety and depression: what are the links?" *J. Clinical Psychiatry,* 62 suppl. 8 (2001): 38–45.

Nemeroff, C.B., "The neurobiology of depression," *Sci. Am.,* 278 (1998): 42–49.

Spiegel, D., "Healing words: emotional expression and disease outcome," *JAMA,* 281 (1999): 1328–1329.

Stam, R., Akkermans, L.M.A., Wiegant, V.M., "Trauma and the gut: interactions between stressful experience and intestinal function," *Gut*, 40 (1997): 704–09.

Walker, E.A., Katon, W.J., Roy-Byrne, P.P., et al., "Histories of sexual victimization in patients with irritable bowel syndrome or inflammatory bowel disease," *Am. J. Psychiatry*, 150 (1993): 1502–06.

Waxman, D., "The irritable bowel: a pathological or a psychological syndrome?" *J. Royal Soc. Med.*, 81 (1988): 718–20.

Weiss, E.L., Longhurst, J.G., Mazure, C.M., "Childhood sexual abuse as a risk factor for depression in women: psychosocial and neurobiological correlates," *Am. J. Psychiatry*, 156 (1999): 541–50.

Whitehead, W.E., Palsson, O.S., "Is rectal pain sensitivity a biological marker for irritable bowel syndrome: psychological influences on pain perception," *Gastroenterology*, 115 (1998): 1263–71.

Chapter 5

Bentley, S.J., Pearson, D.J., Rix, K.J.B., "Food hypersensitivity in irritable bowel syndrome," *The Lancet*, 2 (1983): 295–297.

Bohmer, C.J.M., Tuynman, H.A.R.E., "The effect of a lactose-restricted diet in patients with a positive breath lactose tolerance test, earlier diagnosed as irritable bowel syndrome: a 5-year follow-up study," *Eur. J. Gastroenterol. Hepatol.*, 13 (2001): 941–44.

Bohmer, C.J.M., Tuynman, H.A.R.E., "The clinical relevance of lactose malabsorption in the irritable bowel syndrome," *Eur. J. Gastroenterol. Hepatol.*, 8 (1996): 1013–16.

Bruce, M., Scott, N., Shine, P., et al., "Anxiogenic effects of caffeine in patients with anxiety disorders," *Arch. Gen. Psychiatry*, 49 (1992): 867–69.

Cann, P.A., Read, N.W., Holdsworth, C.D., "What is the benefit of coarse wheat bran in patients with irritable bowel syndrome," *Gut*, 25 (1984): 168–73.

Edwards, R., Peet, M., Shay, J., et al., "Omega-3 polyunsaturated fatty acid levels in the diet and in red blood cell membranes in depressed patients," *J. Affect Disord.* 48 (1998): 149–55.

Eherer, A.H., Porter, J., Fordtran, J.S., "Effect of psyllium, calcium polycarbophil, and wheat bran on secretory diarrhea induced by phenolphthalein," *Gastroenterology*, 104 (1993): 1007–12.

Farah, D.A., Calder, I., Benson, L., et al., "Specific food intolerance: its place as a cause of gastrointestinal symptoms," *Gut*, 26 (1985): 164–168.

Fernandez-Banares, F., Esteve-Pardo, M., de Leon, R., et al., "Sugar malabsorption in functional bowel disease: clinical implications," *American Journal of Gastroenterology,* 88 (1993): 2044–50.

Greden, J.F., Fontaine, P., Lubetsky, M., et al., "Anxiety and depression associated with caffeinism among psychiatric inpatients," *Am. J. Psychiatry,* 135 (1978): 963–66.

Hebden, J.M., Blackshaw, E., D'Amato, M., et al., "Abnormalities of GI transit in bloated irritable bowel syndrome: effect of bran on transit and symptoms," *Am. J. Gastroenterology,* 97 (2002): 2315–20.

Hibbeln, J.R., Salem, N., Jr., "Dietary polyunsaturated fatty acids and depression: when cholesterol does not satisfy," *Am. J. Clin. Nutr.,* 62 (1995): 1–9.

Hotz, J., Plein, K., "Effectiveness of plantago seed husks in comparison with wheat bran on stool frequency and manifestations of irritable colon syndrome with constipation," *Med Kiln,* 89 (1994): 654–51.

Jain, N.K., "Sorbitol intolerance in adults," *American Journal of Gastroenterology,* 80 (1985): 678–81.

Jalihal, A., Kurian, G., "Ispaghula therapy in irritable bowel syndrome: improvement in overall well-being is related to reduction in bowel dissatisfaction," *J. Gastroenterology Hepatology,* 5 (1990): 507–513.

Kawachi, I., Willett, W.C., Colditz, G.A., et al., "A prospective study of coffee drinking and suicide in women," *Arch. Intern. Med.,* 156 (1996): 521–25.

Kellow, J.E., Phillips, S.F., "Altered small bowel motility in irritable bowel syndrome is correlated with symptoms," *Gastroenterology,* 92 (1987): 1885–93.

Maes, M., Christophe, A., Delanghe, J., et al., "Lowered omega-3 polyunsaturated fatty acids in serum phospholipids and cholesterol esters of depressed patients," *Psychiatry Res.,* 85 (1999): 275–91.

Manning, A.P., Heaton, K.W., Harvey, R.F., et al., "Wheat fiber and irritable bowel syndrome," *The Lancet,* (1977): 417–18.

Niec, A.M., Frankum, B., Talley, N.J., "Are adverse food reactions linked to irritable bowel syndrome?" *Am. J. Gastroenterology,* 93 (1998): 2184–90.

Parisi, G.C., Zilli, M., Miani, M.P., et al., "High-fiber supplementation in patients with irritable bowel syndrome (IBS): a multicenter, randomized, open trial comparison between wheat bran and partially hydrolyzed guar gum (PHGG)," *Dig. Disease Science,* 47 (2002): 1697–704.

Pearson, D.J., Bentley, S.J., Rix, K.J.B., et al., "Food hypersensitivity and irritable bowel syndrome," *The Lancet* (1983): 746–747.

Prior, A., Whorwell, P.J., "Double blind study of ispaghula in irritable bowel syndrome," *Gut,* 28 (1987): 1510–13.

Ritchie, J.A., Truelove, S.C., "Comparison of various treatments for irritable bowel syndrome," *Br. J. Med.,* 2 (1980): 1317–19.

Ritchie, J.A., Truelove, S.C., "Treatment of irritable bowel syndrome with lorazepam, hyoscine butylbromide, and ispaghula husk," *Br. Med. J.,* 1 (1979): 376–78.

Sciarretta, G., et al., "Hydrogen breath test quantification and clinical correlation of lactose malabsorption in adult irritable bowel syndrome and ulcerative colitis," *Dig. Dis. Sci.,* 29 (1984): 1098–1104.

Chapter 6

Coppen, A., Chaudrhy, S., Swade, C., "Folic acid enhances lithium prophylaxis," *J. Affect Disorders,* 10 (1986): 91–13.

Dew, M.J., Evans, B.K., Rhodes, J., "Peppermint oil for the irritable bowel syndrome: a multicenter trial," *Br. J. Clin. Practice,* 38 (1984): 394–98.

Di Palma, C., Urani, R., Agricola, R., et al., "Is methylfolate effective in relieving major depression in chronic alcoholics? A hypothesis of treatment," *Curr. Ther. Res.* 55 (1994): 559–67.

Freise, J., Kohler, S., "Peppermint oil/caraway oil – fixed combination in non-ulcer dyspepsia – comparison of the effects of enteric preparations," *Pharmazie,* 54 (1999): 210–15.

Garland, M.L., Hagmeyer, K.O., "The role of zinc lozenges in the treatment of the common cold," *Annals of Pharmacotherapy* 32 (1998): 63–69.

Gee, M.I., Grace, M.G., Wensel, R.H., et al., "Nutritional status of gastroenterology outpatients: comparison of inflammatory bowel disease with functional disorders," *J. Am. Diet Assoc.,* 85 (1985): 1591–99.

Hills, J.M., Aaronson, P.I., "The mechanism of action of peppermint oil on gastrointestinal smooth muscle," *Gastroenterology,* 101 (1991): 55–65.

Ledochowski, M., Murr, C., Lass-Florl, C., et al., "Increased serum amylase and lipase in fructose malabsorbers," *Clin. Chim. Acta,* 311 (2001): 119–23.

Liu, J.H., Chen, G.H., Yeah, H.Z., et al., "Enteric-coated peppermint-oil capsules in the treatment of irritable bowel syndrome: a prospective, randomized trial," *J. Gastroenterology,* 32 (1997): 765–68.

Madisch, A., Melderis, H., Mayr, G., et al., "A plant extract and its modified preparation in functional dyspepsia: results of a double-blind placebo controlled comparative study," *Z. Gastroenterol,* 39 (2001): 511–17.

May, B., Kuntz, H.D., Kieser, M., et al., "Efficacy of a fixed peppermint oil/caraway oil combination in non-ulcer dyspepsia," *Drug Res.,* 46 (1996): 1149–53.

Nobaek, S., Johansson, M.L., Molin, G., et al., "Alteration of intestinal microflora is associated with reduction in abdominal bloating and pain in patients with irritable bowel syndrome," *Am. J. Gastroenterology*, 95 (2000): 1231–38.

Pimentel, M., Chow, E.J., Lin, H.C., "Eradication of small intestinal bacteria overgrowth reduces symptoms of irritable bowel syndrome," *Am. J. Gastroenterology*, 95 (2000): 3503–06.

Reynolds E.H., Preece J.M., Bailey J., et al., "Folic acid, aging, depression, and dementia," *BMJ* 2002; 324:1512–15.

Saavedra, J., "Probiotics and infectious diarrhea," *Am. J. Gastroenterology*, 95 (2000): S16–18.

Chapter 7

Bensoussan, A., Talley, N., Hing, M., et al., "Treatment of irritable bowel syndrome with Chinese herbal medicine: a randomized controlled trial," *JAMA*, 280 (1998): 1585:1589.

Bensoussan, A., "Establishing evidence for Chinese medicine: a case example of irritable bowel syndrome," *Chinese Medical Journal*, 64 (2001): 487–492.

Blanchard, E.B., Greene, B., Scharff, L., et al., "Relaxation training as a treatment for irritable bowel syndrome," *Biofeedback Self Regul.*, 18 (1993): 125–32.

Blanchard, E.B., Schwarz, S.P., Suis, J.M., et al., "Two controlled evaluations of multicomponent psychological treatment of irritable bowel syndrome," *Behav. Res. Ther.*, 30 (1992): 175–189.

Boyce, P., Gilchrist, J., Talley, N.J., et al., "Cognitive-behavioral group therapy as a treatment for irritable bowel syndrome," *Aust. N.Z. J. Psychiatry*, 34 (2000): 300–309.

Braunwald, E., Fauci, A.S., Kasper, D.L., et al., *Harrison's Principles of Internal Medicine*. 15th Edition. (New York: McGraw-Hill, 2001), 249.

DeRubeis, R.J., Gelfand, L.A., Tang, T.Z., et al., "Medications versus cognitive behavior therapy for severely depressed," *Am. J. Psychiatry*, 156 (1999): 1007–13.

Diehl D.L., "Acupuncture for gastrointestinal and hepatobiliary disorders," *J Altern Complement Med* 1999; 5:27-45.

Ernst, E., "Complementary therapies for asthma: what patients use," *Journal of Asthma* 35 (1998): 667–671.

Han, J.S., "Electroacupuncture: an alternative to antidepressants for treating affective disorders," *In. J. Neurosci.*, 29 (1986): 79–92.

Jorm A.F., Christensen H., Griffiths K.M., et al., "Effectiveness of complimentary and self help-treatments for depression," *Med J Aust* 2002; 176:S84–96.

Lamontagne, Y., Annable, L., "Acupuncture and anxiety," *Can. J. Psych.,* 24 (1979): 584–85.

Lin Y., Zhou Z., Shen W., et al., "Clinical and experimental studies on shallow needing technique for treated childhood diarrhea," *J Tradit Chin Med* 1993; 13: 107–14.

Lo, C.W., Chung, Q.Y., "The sedative effect of acupuncture," *Am. J. Chin. Med.,* 7 (1979): 253–259.

Luo, H., Meng, F., Jai, Y., et al., "Clinical research on the therapeutic effect of the electroacupuncture treatment in patients with depression," *Psychiatry Clin. Neurosci.,* 52 (1998): S338–40.

Manber R, Allen J.J., Morris J.J., "Alternative treatments for depression: empirical support and relevance to woman," *J Clin Psychiatry* 2002; 63: 628–40.

Prior, A., Colgan, S.M., Whorwell, P.J., "Changes in rectal sensitivity after hypnotherapy in patients with irritable bowel syndrome," *Gut,* 31 (1990): 896–98.

Roschke, J., Wolf, C., Kogel, P., et al., "Adjuvant whole body acupuncture in depression," *Nervenarzt,* 69 (1998): 961–7.

Smart, H.L., Mayberry, J.F., Atkinson, M., "Alternative medicine consultations and remedies in patients with irritable bowel syndrome," *Gut,* 27 (1986): 826–8.

Thomas, K.B., "General practice consultations: is there any point in being positive?" *British Medical Journal of Clinical Research and Education,* 294 (1987): 1200–1202.

van Dulmen, A.M., Fennis, J.F., Bleijenberg, G., "Cognitive-behavioral group therapy for irritable bowel syndrome: effects and long-term follow-up," *Psychosomatic Medicine,* 58 (1996): 508–14.

Waxman, D., "The irritable bowel: a pathological or a psychological syndrome?" *J. Royal Soc. Med.,* 81 (1988): 718–20.

Whorwell, P.J., Prior, A., Colgan, S.M., "Hypnotherapy in severe irritable bowel syndrome: further experience," *Gut,* 28 (1987): 423–25.

Whorwell, P.J., Prior, A., Faragher, E.S., "Controlled trial of hypnotherapy in the treatment of severe refractory irritable bowel syndrome," *The Lancet,* 2 (1984): 1232–34.

Chapter 8

Colwell, L.J., Prather, C.M., Phillips, S.F., et al., "Effects of an irritable bowel syndrome educational class on health-promoting behaviors and symptoms," *Am. J. Gastroenterology,* 93 (1998): 901–95.

Lustyk, M.K., Jarrett, M.E., Bennett, J.C., et al., "Does a physically active lifestyle improve symptoms in women with irritable bowel syndrome?" *Gastroenterol Nursing,* 24 (2001): 129–37.

Nakaji, S., Tokunaga, S., Sakamoto, J., et al., "Relationship between lifestyle factors and defecation in a Japanese population," *Eur. J. Nutr.,* 41 (2002): 244–48.

Peters, H.P., De Vries, W.R., Vanberge-Henegouwen, G.P., et al., "Potential benefits and hazards of physical activity and exercise on the gastrointestinal tract," *Gut,* 48 (2001): 435–39.

Simren, M., "Physical activity and the gastrointestinal tract," *Eur. J. Gastroenterol Hepatol.,* 14 (2002): 1053–56.

Chapter 9

Ballenger, J.C., Davidson, J.T., Lecrubier, Y., et al., "Consensus statement on depression, anxiety, and functional gastrointestinal disorders," *J. Clin. Psychiatry,* 62 suppl. 8 (2001): 48–51.

Coffin B., Farmachidi J.P., Rueegg P., et al., "Tegaserod, a 5-HT receptor partial agonist, decreases sensitivity to rectal distention in healthy subjects," *Aliment Pharmacol Ther* 2003; 17: 577–85.

Efremova, I., Asnis, G., "Antidepressants in depressed patients with irritable bowel syndrome," *Am. J. Psychiatry,* 155 (1998): 1627–28.

Emmanuel, N.P., Lydiard, R.B., Crawford, M., "Treatment of irritable bowel syndrome with fluvoxamine," *Am. J. Psychiatry,* 154 (1998): 711–12.

Feldman, M., Scharschmidt, B.F., Sleisenger, M.H., *Sleisenger & Fordtran's Gastrointestinal and Liver Disease.* 6th Edition. (New York: W.B. Saunders, 1998) 1545.

Gorard, D.A., Libby, G.W., Farthing, M.J.G., "Effect of a tricyclic antidepressant on small intestinal motility in health and diarrhea-predominant irritable bowel syndrome," *Dig. Dis. Sci.,* 40 (1995): 86–95.

Greenbaum, D.S., Mayle, J.E., Vanegeren, L.E., et al., "Effects of desipramine on irritable bowel syndrome compared with atropine and placebo," *Dig. Dis. Sci.,* 32 (1987): 257–66.

Horwitz, B.J., Fisher, R.S., "The irritable bowel syndrome," *N. Engl. J. Med.,* 344 (2001): 1846–1850.

Hovdenak, N., "Loperamide treatment of the irritable bowel syndrome," *Scand. J. Gastroenterology,* 130 (1987): 81–84

Jailwala, J., Imperiale, T.F., Kroenke, K., "Pharmacologic treatment of the irritable bowel syndrome: a systematic review of the randomized, controlled trials," *Ann. Int. Med.,* 133 (2000): 136–47.

Lydiard, R.B., "Irritable bowel syndrome, anxiety and depression: what are the links?" *J. Clinical Psychiatry,* 62 (2001): S8:38–45.

Muller-Lissner, S.A., Fumagalli, I., Bardhan, K.D., et al., "Tegaserod, a 5-HT(4) receptor partial agonist, relieves symptoms in irritable bowel syndrome patients with abdominal pain, bloating, and constipation," *Aliment Pharmacol. Ther.,* 15 (2001): 1655–66.

Poynard, T., Naveau, S., Mory, B., et al., "Meta-analysis of smooth muscle relaxants in the treatment of irritable bowel syndrome," *Ailment Pharmacol. Ther.,* 8 (1994): 499–510.

Poynard, T., Regimbeau, C., Benhamou, Y., "Meta-analysis of smooth muscle relaxants in the treatment of irritable bowel syndrome," *Aliment Pharmachol. Ther.* 15 (2001): 355–361.

Rajagopalan, M., Kurian, G., Jacob, J., "Symptom relief with amitriptyline in the irritable bowel syndrome," *J. Gastroenterol Hepatol* 13 (1998): 738–41.

Van Outryve, M., Milo, R., Toussaint, J., et al., "Prokinetic treatment of constipation-predominant irritable bowel syndrome: a placebo-controlled study of cisapride," *J. Clin. Gastroenterology,* 13 (1991): 49–57.

Index